Zero
Point

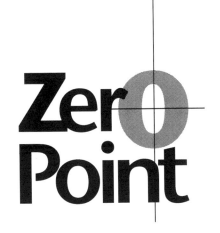

Where Worlds Collide
and
Autism is Born

Betsy Hendricks M.D.

ISBN: 1496181425
ISBN 13: 9781496181428
Library of Congress Control Number: 2014904773
CreateSpace Independent Publishing Platform
North Charleston, South Carolina

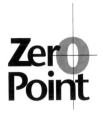

Table of Contents

Gratitude

There are some people, to whom I can never say, "Thank You" enough. Some had the "pleasure" of listening to my ideas and talking with me about all the things I was learning about. Some people were readers who made valuable suggestions regarding readability and content. I was guided through the process of obtaining images that were blended for the cover art. I can read a medical text but was stumped by all the graphic terms when faced with choosing file types and sizes.

The topics in this book have provided material for some lively discussions in clinic. I would never have learned all that I have, if I had not been willing to listen to my patients as they shared what they were learning about. In the work that I do, my patients often become research assistants.

So, "Thank You", to: Amanda, April, Carrie, Heather, Lisa, Merewyn and Paul. "Thank You" to all of my patients that have been a part of my continuing education over the years.

Preface: *Can we find our way back to health?*

Biomedical - When speaking about autism, **biomedical treatment** is a term used to describe a method of evaluation and treatment. It is based on the idea that the symptoms of autism are caused by a medical illness.

This book is my compilation of clues regarding the root cause of autism and treatments to support recovery. This book is about the **biomedical treatment** of autism. This book is, however, about many of today's illnesses, in addition to autism.

The epidemic of autism is increasing. Middle aged people are getting "old people" diseases. Children are dying of rare cancers.

What is going on? Let's look for our first clue. I found this clue in the deep blue sea.

The Deep Blue Sea

People enjoy watching the orca whales of Puget Sound. Whale Watching has become a popular activity and people travel great distances to be able to watch these majestic animals in their native environment. Many of the whales have been named and families of whales are tracked and monitored. It brings us closer to the natural world when we watch these graceful creatures swim and interact. A casual observer might never guess what has been happening to these deep sea neighbors. Do *you* know what is happening to their babies?

What happens to the firstborn calf of an orca whale?

In many cases, the firstborn orca calf dies.

All of these orcas are contaminated with some amount of Polychlorinated Biphenyls (PCBs). PCBs, are members of a family of man-made chemicals called *chlorinated hydrocarbons*. The PCBs enter the water through spills, leaks, damage to equipment and improperly disposed trash.

The production of PCBs was banned in 1979 in the U.S. but the chemical is still in the environment.

PCBs are extremely fat-soluble, meaning they accumulate easily in fats. PCBs in the Puget Sound orcas come from their diet of Chinook salmon which have accumulated PCBs in their fat.

PCBs:
- lower orcas' immunity to diseases.
- decrease sperm count.
- disrupt many hormonal, developmental and reproductive processes.

Once in the orca, the toxins don't go away. These toxins build up in the fatty blubber of the orcas. As PCB concentration increases, it severely decreases the orca's lifespan.

Can any of the orcas decrease their level of PCBs?

Only sexually mature females have a chance of getting rid of any PCBs. While pregnant, some of the PCBs transfer to the developing offspring. After birth, even more toxins are transferred to the baby when excreted through the mother's breast milk which is extremely rich in fat.

Having offspring increases the mother's chance of survival.

Studies show female blubber samples have one-third the levels of PCB toxins found in male orcas. Having offspring increases the mothers chance of survival.

However, the PCB levels in the developing calf, especially the first-born, often lead to its premature death.

It sometimes takes multiple attempts for female orcas to have a calf with low enough PCB levels to survive.[1][2][3]

Should we care about what is happening to the orcas?

Well, yes, I think we should. Actually, on many levels, we should care about what is happening to the orcas. As our deep sea neighbors, we should care about their health and well-being. As a reflection of what is happening to our own children, we should care about the tragedy unfolding. You see, chlorinated molecules such as PCBs are amazing things, and not in a good way. These are new, human-created molecules that may have appeared to solve other problems, but have wreaked havoc through multiple ecosystems and food webs, including our own. In the end, these and other modern chemicals have caused significant new problems.

The health crisis of the orcas gives us clues about our own current health crisis.

I am writing this book from the perspective of a doctor, a mother, and a grandmother. I have worked with families in clinic and as I watched my grandsons grow and develop, I realized that no family is exempt from the current health crisis.

Every child does not have autism, but every child is at risk for developmental and/or chronic disorders. We are seeing a significant increase in the number of children with:
- allergies
- ear infections
- asthma
- learning disorders
- behavior disorders
- developmental delays
- speech delay
- ADD/ADHD
- autism
- cancer
- auto-immune diseases

It is not our imagination and it is getting worse, not better.
Can we stop this trend and turn things around?

I think we can. Let's look at our clues and the evidence that is available in the scientific and medical literature. Let's start with "Biomedical".

Biomedical

I use the biomedical approach for children with autism spectrum disorders, and for just about anyone with a modern, chronic illness.

You may have been told that there is no treatment for children with autism. You may have been told that there is no evidence that biomedical treatment can be helpful. You may have talked with families who are "doing biomedical" and have learned otherwise.

To understand some of the controversy regarding whether biomedical treatments work, it is helpful to understand some of our history in the medical field.

In our medical training, we learned that there are many illnesses that are idiopathic.

Idiopathic - an illness with an unknown cause.

Any time we learned about treating an idiopathic illness, we were taught that the cause is unknown and the best we can do is to treat symptoms and try to keep it from getting worse.

We were taught that the many illnesses were idiopathic and could not be reversed, including:
• High blood pressure
• Diabetes, type II
• Heart disease

I have since learned that many illnesses can be successfully reversed. As I get a better understanding of what is causing an illness, I am better able to understand how to reverse the disease process.

As we develop a better understanding of the underlying cause, the root, of an illness, we better understand how to actually treat that illness.

Let me give you an example. Let's talk about scurvy.

Back in the time of world exploration on sailing ships, sailors would get sick with an illness called scurvy. It was an idiopathic illness. No one knew what caused it. Eventually, it was discovered that if citrus fruit was included in the diet on the voyages, scurvy could be avoided.

We now know that scurvy is due to a lack of vitamin C. Now that we know the cause, it is easy to prevent and can even be treated.

Join me on a clue finding expedition.

Throughout this book, we will be looking at clues related to the root cause of autism and other chronic illnesses.

Introduction: User Information

What follows on these pages, is an account of my thought processes and experiences.

This is not specific medical advice.

I have provided the information for you to use with your own health care team.

Chapter 1:

Zero Point

I love a mystery. I love puzzles. I thought a murder mystery game was the only mystery I would ever participate in solving. Wouldn't it be fun to dress in character and try to figure out "who done it?"?

I still might do that one of these days. For now, I've got a bigger mystery to solve, and the players in this game are dangerous and deadly.

What is this mystery?
The mystery is, "Why are we having this exploding epidemic of autism and other childhood illnesses?"

Why do I care?
I care because this affects virtually every family I know. This affects my family. If you are reading this book, I am guessing that this affects your family.

The clues. Follow the clues.
Throughout this book, we will be looking at clues. Then, we will be looking at how these clues all tie together. Perhaps, by using

this information, and sharing this information, we can put the brakes on this out-of-control train and keep it from going over the cliff.

What out-of-control train? The mystery begins! Let's look at some clues.

I am going to mix my metaphors just a little here. Image a comfortable train ride. You have been planning a vacation and have tickets to "FamilyLand". Everything seems fine on the train. The food looks perfect and tastes wonderful. You appreciate the subtle fragrance from the air fresheners. The complimentary lotion makes your skin feels soft and it also has a gentle fragrance. The bathrooms have antibacterial soaps and you can still smell the disinfecting cleaners that were used. Everything on this trip is convenient and comfortable. There are no immediate problems associated with your environment.

What could go wrong?

But, as you ride on this train, you notice that the children begin behaving differently. Some are aggressive. Some are screaming. Some have stopped talking. Some simply sit and rock back and forth. Some are having seizures. Some are even dying, right before your eyes.

Then, it is not only the children that are affected. You see the older individuals on the train begin to talk nonsense. They can't remember what you said to them 2 minutes ago. Middle-aged people are noticing that they hurt all over and are having difficulty concentrating. Young people are having heart attacks and then, they are gone. (Does any of this sound eerily familiar?)

It's almost like everyone has been poisoned on this train. Actually, it is exactly like everyone has been poisoned on this train. But, everything looked so pretty and comfortable, no one believed it could be happening.

What happened?

What if I told you that the "food" on the train is a conglomeration of chemicals (many toxic) with an abundant amount of sugar and salt so that it has some flavor.

What if I told you that the agricultural chemicals used in growing the base material for the "food" are toxic to your cells and interfere with insulin sensitivity.

What if I told you that the chemicals in the air freshener are interfering with your liver's ability to clear other toxins.

What if I told you that the complimentary lotion and the antibacterial soap are providing additional toxins and endocrine disruptors that you absorb right through your skin.

If I told you all of these things, would you begin to understand why everyone on the train is getting sick? Would you begin to understand why so many people on this planet are getting sick?

Endocrine Disruptor - a chemical that PRETENDS to be one (or more) of your own hormones and either interferes with these hormones or overly mimics the hormones.

Who is affected by these toxins?

Let's look again at our train. More and more people are getting sick, and now, the doctors and other scientists on-board this train, are wondering if anyone will still be alive by the time the train arrives in "FamilyLand".

I'm on this train and so are you. We have to figure out what is going on. Where do we begin?

Where do we begin in order to figure out what is going on?

Let's take the first step to solve this mystery.

Let's start with some information that is generally accepted about autism. Many people agree that it is a combination of genetic factors, environmental factors, and possibly nutrient deficiencies, that are contributing to our epidemic of autism. Let's take a closer look at these three factors in a Venn Diagram.

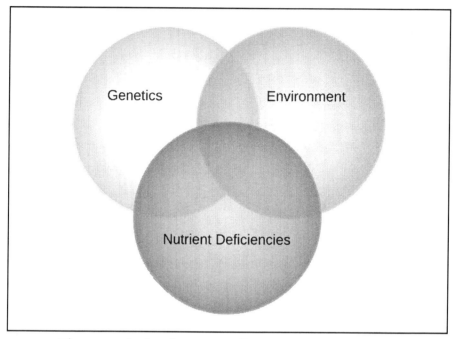

The association between Genetics, Environment and Nutrient Deficiencies.

Venn Diagram - A Venn Diagram illustrates the relationship between 2 or more sets of information. You find common elements in the areas where the circles overlap. I use the Venn Diagram to show where interactions can occur between the sets.

Autism and this Venn Diagram.
You may be familiar with this Venn Diagram. This is the one many of us have seen for years, showing the intersection, or overlap, of these three major factors:
- GENETIC PREDISPOSITION
- ENVIRONMENTAL FACTORS
- NUTRIENT DEFICIENCIES

This diagram helps to explain the epidemic of autism. This diagram actually helps to explain the explosion of chronic illnesses, including obesity, that we are seeing in adults and children.

Journey to the Center of the Venn diagram!

We are going to travel to the center of this Venn Diagram. I am calling the center of this Venn Diagram the "Zero Point". At the "Zero Point", I see a specific cellular mechanism that is affected by Genetics, Environment, and by Nutrient Deficiencies. This is what I see from my perspective. This may not be what you see. This may not be what many of my fellow physicians see.

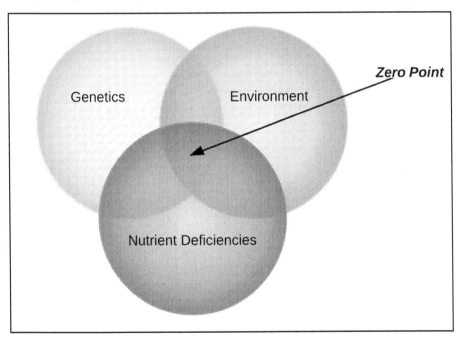

"Zero Point": I see a specific cellular mechanism that is affected by Genetics, Environment, and by Nutrient Deficiencies.

At the center of the Venn Diagram, I see a cellular mechanism that is influenced by these three major factors. This cellular mechanism involves insulin.

What role does insulin have in autism?

I was looking for something to explain "the blank look"; that stare that develops after regression. I was looking for an explanation of the aggression, the meltdowns, the anxiety and the terror.

The more I learned about insulin and glucose regulation in the brain, the more I saw that this could be related to the symptoms we see in autism.

The more I learned about factors that disrupt insulin and glucose regulation, the more I saw the relationship to autism and other chronic illnesses.

A "theory of everything" for autism.

Physicists are looking for the unifying "theory of everything" that will explain how the universe works - from the action of subatomic particles, to gravity, to dark matter and black holes. They have developed a "theory of almost everything" but it is incomplete. It does not include gravity or dark matter.

I am sure my "Zero Point" is also incomplete. However, we cannot stop striving to complete our own "theory of everything" that leads to autism. The lives of our children and future generations depends on our unrelenting quest to build on the accumulating data that we use to create our model of Autism.

Model of Autism.

Our model should ideally explain:
1. The influence of gluten sensitivity.
2. The influence of heavy metal exposure (including mercury) and air pollution.
3. The influence of brain injury (which includes encephalitis).

4. The influence of mother's toxic burden.
5. The influence of medications and vaccinations.
6. The influence of deficiency of vitamin B12.
7. The influence of vitamin B6.
8. The 4 (almost 5):1 ratio of boys to girls affected.
9. The role of genetics - why doesn't every child have autism?

Our model should show the relationship of these things to autism, as well as to the "Zero Point". Many of these influences have a genetic component and/or an environmental influence and/or is influenced by nutritional deficiencies.

When my children were small, there was a cartoon about a "scientist" who every day planned to "take over the world!" Let's pretend to be a "mad scientist" for a few minutes, and build a machine to create "Autism".

Building a Model of Autism.

Step 1. Build a machine with 3 sliding switches named: Genetics, Environment, Nutritional Deficiencies. When the switch is all the way to the left, the value is ZERO. When the switch is all the way to the right, the value is 10.

Step 2. Build the internal circuits, so that when the value of the 3 switches adds up to a critical level (in this case, use "10" as the value), a light will flash.

When the combination of genetics, environment and nutritional deficiencies adds up to a critical level, Autism can occur.

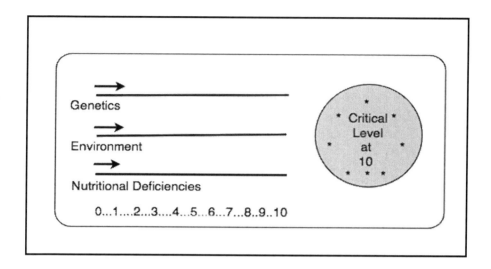

In the cases of autism mostly associated with genetics (this is in the next chapter, where I talk about genetics and autism), the switch for Genetics would be at a value of 10. The other switches may or may not be shifted to the right.

In the cases of autism that are influenced by 2 or 3 of the "switches", then any combination that adds up to 10 would cause our model to light up. So, even someone with "good genes" could be affected by a toxic load of "10", or by a combination of a toxic load of "3" and nutrient deficiencies of "7".

What if we slide the switches back to the left?

Can we slide the switches back to the left? We cannot change the genes we are born with, but research is showing that we can change the expression of many of our genes. The field of epigenetics is helping to explain how people are reversing many illnesses, such as Multiple Sclerosis, previously thought to be irreversible!

We are learning how to change our environment so that we can move that switch to the left.

Nutritional deficiencies can be identified and treated which will move that switch to the left.

We can learn to move ALL the switches back towards the left.

What do we know about moving the switches towards the left?

We have years of research by clinicians, research scientists and parents (yes - parents!) that have demonstrated some interventions that are beneficial. These interventions influence all three of the switches in the model.

As I build and revise my working model of autism, I look at how the interventions that help our children (and us) recover have influenced the "Zero Point". As I build and revise my working model of autism, I look at how the "Zero Point" is related to autism and other chronic disease states.

These interventions include (but are not limited to):

1. Removal of heavy metals.
2. Gluten-free/Casein-free diet.
3. Low-inflammatory diet/Autoimmune diet (SCD, GAPS, Paleo).
4. Low Histamine diet.
5. Glutathione and nutrients that support glutathione production.
6. Charcoal and/or Bentonite Clay.
7. Vitamin B12.
8. Vitamin B6.
9. Folate.
10. Fats (Omega3s, saturated fats)
11. Vitamin D.
12. Probiotics and restoring health of GI tract.
13. Iodine.

SCD - Specific Carbohydrate Diet.

GAPS - Gut and Psychology Syndrome diet.

Paleo - A Paleo-type diet is patterned after what scientist are determining humans ate prior to the domestication of grains. The scientist have looked for clues associating diet with optimal health. The diet emphasizes nutrient dense foods that have the least amount of inflammatory properties. Coincidentally (or not) this type of diet is very similar to the healing-type diets that have been developed in the past, such as SCD and GAPS.

These diets are further refined based on individual food sensitivities and level of inflammation.

It's a process.

Helping my patients find their way to health and wellness is a process. It is a "Spiral Path to Wellness", not a straight line to the finish line.

Finding my way to the "Zero Point" has been a process. (Yes, Belinda, put it on my tombstone - "It's a Process"!)

I see patterns. In my mind, I make models of interacting variables. I read studies and collect information. I love mysteries and solving puzzles. My undergraduate degree was in biology, but my minors were computer science, mathematics and physical science.

I observe my patients in clinic and listen to the family stories. I work with individuals and families, teaching and learning, to survive in a world gone mad with technological advances that have unforeseen outcomes.

Is it yeast?

When I first began studying the biomedical evaluation and treatment of autism, I realized that, for many individuals, yeast appeared to play a significant role in the illness. The children had yeast and symptoms associated with yeast. Often, the mother had a chronic yeast problem. Yeast appeared to be a significant factor for many patients. Sometimes, symptoms would improve when a "yeast diet" was followed, even if the lab testing failed to show evidence of yeast. Sometimes, symptoms would improve with probiotic treatment. Was yeast causing the illness? Was biofilm involved?

Yeast - Yeast are microorganisms that are part of the Fungi kingdom. Yeast are a normal component of the microflora of the human body. The microflora is primarily composed of yeast and bacteria. The microflora is found in the GI tract and on the surface of the body.

Is it biofilm?
Studying the role of biofilm helped to explain how the yeast could escape laboratory detection while still causing symptoms and illness. However, the role of yeast in the illness could only explain a part of what we are seeing. I knew there had to be more.

Biofilm - Microorganisms that have adhered to a surface and are within a polymeric substance that they have created. Microorganisms within a biofilm structure may be more resistant to antimicrobial chemicals (such as antibiotics). Microorganisms within a biofilm structure may be more successful at evading the host's immune system.

If not yeast, what is it? Is it a lack of glutathione?
Over the years, as I have learned of the many things that can lead to the illness we call autism, the one common point, the "Zero Point", eluded me. Much can be centered around glutathione and mitochon-drial function, but there was still a key point missing.

Glutathione - Glutathione is an antioxidant. It is the major endogenous antioxidant produced in our cells. It can neutralize free radicals and can maintain vitamins C and E (these are also antioxidants) in their active forms. Glutathione is used in many reactions in the cells. Every system in the body can be affected by the availability of active glutathione (reduced glutathione).

What is this "Zero Point" where the 3 circles overlap?
One day, while reading yet another article, I saw it. Maybe it is all circumstantial, but it adds to my working model and, for now, seems to make sense.
　　The "Zero Point" appears to be related to insulin resistance.

I have found a lot of evidence that relates to this "Zero Point" and to my working model of autism. A lot of "we have evidence of" and "this study shows". Don't get me wrong, these are all very important. If we didn't have evidence to give us information to build this model with, there would be no model at all.

Searching for clues.
I began digging for more clues and more links to the "Zero Point". The more I dug, the more I uncovered links and a trail of clues that led, not only to the now "known" risk factors for autism, but also to the Biomedical interventions that have been used with different levels of success since Dr. Bernard Rimland first saw a link to vitamin B6 in the 1970s.

Pointing treatment interventions at the "Zero Point".
The "Zero Point" may provide us with a new working framework for our Biomedical treatment of the *systemic illness* that produces the behaviors and characteristics we call **autism**. In this book, we are also going to look at the next question, perhaps an even bigger question, of "What causes this 'Zero Point' to occur?"

What causes this "Zero Point" to occur and can it be switched on and off?
I am a first generation child of post-World War II parents. My daughters are in the second generation, and my grandchildren are third generation children. I did not fully realize the significance of this until I saw the "switch" flip.

What switch? Is this related to the "Zero Point"?
I know many parents have seen the "switch" flip, with seeing their child "there" one day, and then changed, with loss of eye-contact, loss of speech, onset of screaming and aggression, within 24 hours.

In many cases, this "switch" flipped at the time of some specific vaccinations.

I saw a switch in the other direction, with a restoration occurring within 24 hours. Alas, this change was not initially permanent, but gave us a glimpse into what could be and how to get there. Where did this switch come from? To answer this question, we have to have a short history lesson.

How World War II changed the world.

World War II is significant for a variety of reasons. It was after this war that "Better Living through Chemistry" really took off. Factories that had been involved in producing weapons (and chemicals) of war, now looked to other sectors of the marketplace.[4] The oil industry had produced fuel for fast cars, and byproducts of the gasoline industry were finding their way into *every* segment of our lives.

Many of the chemical byproducts have allowed cheaper products to be produced in the food industry, the farm industry, the body-care product industry and in household cleaning product industry. We have ingredients in our food that are not allowed in much of the rest of the civilized world. Toxins that have been banned in this country since the 1970s are still present in the environment and in the food web. There are toxins in make-up and body-care products that are absorbed through our skin and persist for years. These are toxins that are associated with cancer and chronic disease.

With each successive generation since World War II, we are seeing an increase in chronic disease and an explosion in the rates of childhood illnesses, including autism.

Is this a coincidence?

We are going to follow the clues and see what leads to the "Zero Point" and how this relates to autism.

Chapter 2:

Model of Autism

Building a working model for autism.

I'm going to walk you through this version of my working model, step by step. Let's start with the Venn Diagram first. The famous (famous in the Autism Research Institute and the AutismOne world) Venn Diagram that shows the overlap of Genetic Predisposition, Environmental Factors, and Nutrient Deficiencies.

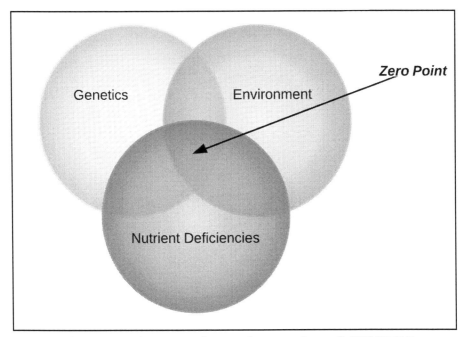

This Venn diagram shows the overlap of GENETIC PREDISPOSITION, ENVIRONMENTAL FACTORS, and NUTRIENT DEFICIENCIES.

Genetics and detoxification ability.

For the purpose of building this model, I think of GENETIC PREDISPOSITION in terms of how well a person can detoxify.

Detoxify - To break down chemicals into less harmful substances and/or eliminate chemicals from the body.

How much toxic material can your system clear in a day?

The ability to detoxify varies from person to person. The ability to detoxify depends on two major variables.

1. How large a VOLUME of toxins can be dealt with in a single unit of time (minute, hour, day).
2. Which of the different TYPES of toxins can be cleared efficiently.

In other words, just how much toxin can you clear in a day? And, can you clear all the toxins you are exposed to?

Super detoxifiers are people that are the least affected by our toxic world.

Some people are great detoxifiers. They can walk through a toxic waste dump and feel fine. They can eat just about anything and feel fine. They can run and run and run, and still have energy. They are the least likely to be affected by the environmental factors.

People with Multiple Chemical Sensitivity (MCS) may have a decreased ability to detoxify.

At the other end of the spectrum are those who are the least able to detoxify. Some of these people will develop multiple chemical sensitivities. When they pump gas into their car, they have a metallic taste in their mouth. Their detoxification pathways are slow. They can't clear the toxins as fast as their exposure. They fatigue easily. They are not marathon runners. They can hardly get out of their chair. They haven't been able to efficiently clear toxins and their cells are poisoned.

Many people with multiple chemical sensitivities will have lab testing that appears to be normal. As a result, many have been "dismissed" as having no illness at all. However, organic acid and amino acid testing may show impaired ability to detoxify, as well as an increase in nutrient need.

Babies have the least ability to detoxify.

The detoxification systems in a baby do not have the same capacity as an adult. Is it any wonder that children are our "canaries in the coal mine"? A baby can only detoxify a fraction of the amount that an adult can detoxify.

Glutathione is a clue. Glutathione is the great detoxifier.

Where a person falls on the detoxification spectrum depends on several factors. Part of this has to do with methylation (may be influenced by an MTHFR mutation) and glutathione production.

Part of this has to do with other detoxification pathways within the cells and the genes that code for the enzymes involved in these pathways. There is NOT A SINGLE GENE that is responsible. It is a COMBINATION OF GENES that code for a number of enzymes that are involved in detoxification.

Methylation - the addition of a methyl group to a molecule. A methyl group is CH3 (one carbon atom with 3 hydrogen atoms).

Glutathione - a molecule that is a major antioxidant and also is involved in detoxification of chemicals.

Are you a great detoxifier?

People who have a lower capacity for detoxification are more likely to be poisoned by toxins in our environment. This is part of the reason that some people are affected, and some are not. This helps to explain why some children have autism, and some do not.

Genetics, insulin and glutamate receptors.

There is another Genetic Predisposition that appears to also be involved in the development of autism. This involves the PI3K/Tor pathway. This pathway is the major pathway for insulin signals within cells. There is evidence that hyperactivation of this pathway leads to increased sensitivity to induction by glutamate receptors. [5] Hyperactivation of this pathway occurs with elevated levels of insulin as seen in Insulin Resistance.

Translation - *There is an association between insulin resistance and glutamate receptors.*

Glutamate receptors are important for learning and memory formation. Glutamate is an excitatory neurotransmitter. GABA, which is made from glutamate, is an inhibitory (calming) neurotransmitter.

Genetics and autism.

There are some specific, genetic-linked disorders with a higher frequency of autism and autism spectrum disorders. These include Tuberous sclerosis, type I Neurofibromatosis, and autism with macrocephaly. Also, Fragile X is associated with a higher frequency of autism and autism spectrum disorders.

These disorders all share a common characteristic. In each of these disorders, there are genes that code for enzymes that *interfere with inhibition* of the PI3K/Tor pathway.

Please keep in mind, that virtually every system in the body is built around a system of "checks and balances". One action or activity will "stimulate" and another action or activity will "inhibit". It is the balance of both of these actions that yields the desired effect.

Overstimulation of a pathway that is associated with glutamate receptors.

When we talk about the PI3K/Tor pathway, there are multiple things to "stimulate" the pathway, and multiple things to "inhibit" the pathway. If you lose some of the inhibition on this pathway, then the result is overstimulation. If you have excessive stimuli (insulin), then the result is overstimulation of this pathway.

Environmental link to the pathway associated with glutamate receptors.

For children who do NOT have one of the listed genetic-linked disorders with a higher frequency of autism and autism spectrum disorders (Tuberous sclerosis, type I Neurofibromatosis, autism with macrocephaly, Fragile X), this pathway may be involved in an ENVIRONMENTAL link to autism.

Environmental factors can lead to overstimulation of the pathway associated with glutamate receptors.

In the case of an ENVIRONMENTAL influence, the genetic abnormality that leads to overactivation of PI3K/Tor is not present. However, there are ENVIRONMENTAL factors that can lead to **hyperinsulinemia** and overstimulation of the PI3K/Tor pathway.

What are these environmental factors?

ENVIRONMENTAL FACTORS include the chemicals that we are exposed to (from the air, water, living and work environment, chemicals on foods) as well as the actual food that we eat. Some of these chemicals are toxins.

When does toxin exposure begin?

Toxin exposure does not begin after birth. Babies are born with a toxic burden. This means that before a baby is ever born, it is exposed to an unbelievable level of toxins that are circulating in the mother. This is not a problem limited to a few mothers. This is very likely happening to just about every mother in the world.

How have we learned about the toxic load of newborns?

The Body Burden Study, commissioned by the Environmental Working Group (EWG), found up to 232 toxic chemicals in the umbilical cord blood of 10 babies. These 10 children were born between December 2007 and June 2008 in Michigan, Florida, Massachusetts, California and Wisconsin.

What was found in the cord blood, in the blood circulating in the babies?

There were 21 contaminants found for the first time in American newborns, including Bisphenol A (BPA). BPA is a synthetic estrogen that disrupts the endocrine system, disrupts normal reproductive system development and diminishes test animals' intellectual and behavioral capacity. The 232 toxic chemicals found in these babies included endocrine disruptors, and neurotoxins.

Ten of ten of the newborns had measurable levels of *lead, mercury, methylmercury and Polychlorinated biphenyls (PCBs).*

Every baby

lead
mercury
methylmercury
polychlorinated biphenyls (PCBs).

Where are these chemicals found in our environment?

According to the EWG, the chemicals found in these babies are from unintended exposures to some of the most problematic consumer product and commercial chemicals ever put on the market. These products are found in our supermarkets and department stores. We have bought these products and brought them into our homes. We have then exposed ourselves by cleaning our homes, washing our bodies and applying body care products to our skin. We have exposed ourselves by consuming toxins in the foods that we eat.

Think back to the out-of-control train from Chapter 1.

Everything seems fine on the train. The food looks perfect and tastes wonderful. You appreciate the subtle fragrance from the air fresheners. The complimentary lotion makes your skin feels soft and it also has a gentle fragrance. The bathrooms have antibacterial soaps and you can still smell the disinfecting cleaners that were used. Everything on this trip is convenient and comfortable. There are no immediate problems associated with your environment.

Where can I find more information about this study?
Please take a few minutes to look at this report. This will help you get an idea of the level of toxins I am talking about. This is about the toxins in your body, your spouse/partner's body, and in each of your children. http://www.ewg.org/research/minority-cord-blood-report/bpa-and-other-cord-blood-pollutants [6]

How were these babies exposed to these chemicals before birth?
All the chemicals found in the newborns had been part of the toxic body burden of the mother. While in the uterus, the mother's detoxification systems are helping to eliminate the toxins from her body and from the baby's body. Once born, the infant's liver has the task of detoxifying chemicals all on its own.

Nutrient deficiencies can affect a person's ability to detoxify.
NUTRIENT DEFICIENCIES can occur due to:
• Environmental Factors.
• Poor nutrition.
• Illnesses caused by Genetics and/or Environmental Factors.
These NUTRIENT DEFICIENCIES, can then, in turn, affect a person's ability to detoxify.

Now that we have built our working model, we have -

A Perfect Storm to create Autism.

So, when talking about the 3 factors in the Venn Diagram, you may be able to see how a "Perfect Storm" of genetic predisposition (decreased ability to detoxify), level of toxic exposure, and nutrient deficiencies, could set a person up for serious disease.

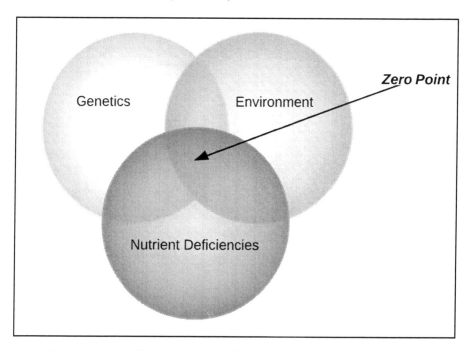

A decreased ability to detoxify (genetics), along with toxins (environment) and lack of key nutrients (nutrient deficiencies) can create a "Perfect Storm" environment and Autism.

Chapter 3:

Clues that Lead to a Cause of Autism

This chapter provides clues and the supporting evidence for those clues. Some of the material can be a challenge to read, even for the scientifically inclined.

The important points are in the bold print. For more in-depth understanding of the points, the supporting evidence and commentary are provided.

Gluten and Autism

A big clue. Gluten.

Ah, gluten. Many parents have been saying for years that they could see improvements when their child began eating a gluten-free diet. However, most of the children did not have Celiac disease. Most of the children I tested in clinic, had gluten sensitivity and did not have the genetic predisposition for Celiac disease. We have learned, in recent years, that there really is a medically defined entity called Gluten Sensitivity. And guess what the scientists have recently discovered. Did you guess it yet?

A study linking gluten sensitivity and autism.

This is from a study published June 18, 2013. In this study, 24.2% of children with autism and 5.3% of controls were positive for having elevated IgG antibodies to gliadin.

"Conclusions. A subset of children with autism displays increased immune reactivity to gluten, the mechanism of which appears to be distinct from that in celiac disease. The increased anti-gliadin antibody response and its association with GI symptoms points to a potential mechanism involving immunologic and/or intestinal permeability abnormalities in affected children." [7]

Translation - Some children with autism have evidence of an immune reaction to gluten. These children may not have celiac disease, but have what we now call Gluten Sensitivity. The immune reaction and the history of GI symptoms suggests involvement of the immune system and/or abnormal intestinal permeability (leaky gut).

Gluten and neurologic disease, not a new idea.

The idea that gluten can be associated with neurologic disease is not completely new. A very interesting editorial was published in 2002, discussing gluten sensitivity as a neurological illness. This editorial contained information from a landmark paper that was published in 1966.

Gluten sensitivity is associated with changes in the Cerebellum.

This paper described 16 patients with Celiac disease and neurological disorders. Ten of these patients had severe progressive neuropathy. All had gait ataxia and some had limb ataxia.

Postmortem examination of tissue showed extensive perivascular inflammatory changes in both the central and peripheral nervous systems. It was noted that a striking feature was the loss of Purkinje cells with atrophy and gliosis of the **cerebellum**. All 16 had evidence of severe malabsorption and vitamin deficiencies.

Ataxia and peripheral neuropathy are neurological manifestations seen in Celiac disease.

Further review of reports from that time onward, showed that ataxia and peripheral neuropathy were the most common neurological manifestations seen in patients with confirmed Celiac disease.

During the 8 years prior to this editorial, the author had been using antigliadin antibodies to screen patients with neurological dysfunction of unknown etiology.

Patients with neurological disease of unknown etiology had higher levels of antigliadin antibodies.

He found that patients with neurological disease of unknown etiology were found to have a much higher prevalence of circulating antigliadin antibodies (57%) in their blood than either the control subjects (12%) or those with neurological disorders of known etiology (5%).

He also noted that it was unlikely that these neurological disorders were a result of nutrient deficiencies as the subjects were rarely deficient in B12, folate, vitamin D or vitamin E. Two-thirds of these patients had no enteropathy (intestinal damage). Postmortem findings from two of his patients with gluten ataxia showed perivascular cuffing with both CD4 and CD8 cells. This inflammation was primarily seen in the white matter of the **cerebellum**. There was also marked Purkinje cell loss. He has also found antibodies against Purkinje cells in patients with gluten ataxia.

His research suggests that IgG antigliadin antibodies cross-react with epitopes on Purkinje cells from human **cerebellum**. (Translation - Antibodies of the immune system attack cells in the **cerebellum**.) [8]

Antigliadin Antibodies - Antibodies, made by the immune system that "attack" gliadin (from gluten) or endogenous molecules (molecules of self) that appear to be similar to the gliadin.

Purkinje cells - A specific type of cell that is only found in the **cerebellum**.

To have a better understanding of gluten and autism, let's spend a little time learning about the cerebellum.

Cerebellum

More clues are found in the structural changes that occur in the cerebellum.

The cerebellum is a part of the brain that helps control balance and motor function, including muscle tone. The cerebellum also has a role in cognitive function, including language.

Cognitive and emotional disorders may either accompany cerebellar diseases, or in some cases, may be the principal clinical presentation.

Behavioral changes may be the primary presenting symptom of cerebellar dysfunction.

Again, just as we see new information emerging regarding gluten sensitivity, we are seeing new information emerging regarding cerebellar function. In the past, it was thought that the cerebellum was primarily responsible for helping control balance and motor function. Now, there is published evidence that behavioral changes may be the primary presenting symptoms.

Children with loss of cerebellar function, either through surgery or absence of part of the cerebellum at birth (congenital), display characteristic behavioral deficits. These deficits include difficulties with speech, irritability, impulsivity, disinhibition, and lability of affect. Some were noted to have autistic-like features.

Surgery affecting the cerebellum is associated with a behavioral syndrome that includes regressive personality changes.
In about 15% of children who undergo resection of midline cerebellar tumors, "posterior fossa syndrome" was noted. In this syndrome, there is dysarthria, apraxia, and a behavioral syndrome that includes regressive personality changes, apathy, withdrawal and poverty of spontaneous movement. There is rapid fluctuation of expression of emotion that gravitates between irritability with inconsolable crying and agitation, to giggling and easy distractibility.

Loss of some or all of the cerebellum can result in gross and fine motor delay, apraxia and ataxia, as well as autistic-like behaviors.
In children with complete or partial absence of cerebellum, children were noted to have gross and fine motor delay, oral motor apraxia, clumsiness and mild ataxia. Behavioral features included autistic-like stereotypical performance, obsessive rituals, and difficulty understanding social cues. Some children have expressive language delay as the principal manifestation. [9]

Dysarthria - In a person with dysarthria, a nerve, brain, or muscle disorder makes it difficult to use or control the muscles of the mouth, tongue, larynx, or vocal cords, which make speech.
The muscles may be weak or completely paralyzed, or it may be difficult for the muscles to work together. [10]
Apraxia - Apraxia is a disorder of the brain and nervous system in which a person is unable to perform tasks or movements when asked, even though:
The request or command is understood
They are willing to perform the task

The muscles needed to perform the task work properly

The task may have already been learned. [11]

Ataxia - failure of muscle control in the arms and legs that result in movement disorders. [12]

Abnormalities in the cerebellum can be associated with the behaviors of autism.

Heavy Metals, Air Pollution and Autism

Are there clues linking heavy metals, such as mercury, to autism? Are there clues linking other chemicals to autism?
There have been numerous studies showing a link between heavy metals and autism. There are also studies showing a link between air pollution and autism.

A link is seen between chlorinated solvents, heavy metals and autism. A look at a dangerous duo.
One study that combines research on heavy metals and air pollution is from the San Francisco Bay Area. This study looked at 19 different hazardous air pollutants. The hazardous air pollutant concentrations were compiled by the United States Environmental Protection Agency.

An association was seen between autism and chlorinated solvents and heavy metals, but not for aromatic solvents. The individual compounds with the highest associations included mercury, cadmium, nickel, trichloroethylene and vinyl chloride.[13]

One thing we might learn from this study is that the combination of chlorinated chemicals and heavy metals is a dangerous duo.

Mice with autoimmune disease were more susceptible to the influence of thimerosal and showed growth delay, behavior changes and altered glutamate receptors.
This study was published in Molecular Psychiatry in 2004. The researchers had 2 sets of mice, each with a different Major Histocompatibility Complex (MHC) gene set. One group, the SJL/J mice, were autoimmune disease-sensitive. The other group, the C57BL/6J and BALB/cJ mice, were not autoimmune disease-sensitive.

The researchers exposed the mice to thimerosal in doses and timing equivalent to the pediatric immunization schedule that was in use in the US in 2001.

Thimerosal - From the FDA website, "Thimerosal is a mercury-containing organic compound (an organomercurial). Since the 1930s, it has been widely used as a preservative in a number of biological and drug products, including many vaccines, to help prevent potentially life threatening contamination with harmful microbes. Over the past several years, because of an increasing awareness of the theoretical potential for neurotoxicity of even low levels of organomercurials and because of the increased number of thimerosal containing vaccines that had been added to the infant immunization schedule, concerns about the use of thimerosal in vaccines and other products have been raised. Indeed, because of these concerns, the Food and Drug Administration has worked with, and continues to work with, vaccine manufacturers to reduce or eliminate thimerosal from vaccines." (http://www.fda.gov/BiologicsBloodVaccines/SafetyAvailability/VaccineSafety/UCM096228)

The SJL/J mice (the autoimmune disease-sensitive mice) showed growth delay; reduced locomotion; exaggerated response to novelty; and densely packed, hyperchromic hippocampal neurons with altered glutamate receptors and transporters. The other mice were not susceptible to the influence of the thimerosal.[14]

A family history of autoimmune disease may be related to the influence of thimerosal and development of autism.

The results of this study could help explain why some children are susceptible to damage from thimerosal while some appear to be resistant to damage from thimerosal. If this translates into humans subjects, then this could explain why, when there is a family history of autoimmune disease, a child could develop autism after having followed the pediatric immunization schedule prior to withdrawal of thimerosal from many vaccines.

Are there still vaccines that contain thimerosal?

Yes. There are still several thimerosal-containing vaccines, with the most commonly administered one being the "flu shot".

Should people with autoimmune disease get the "flu shot"?

They may want to review the risks and benefits of the "flu shot" first.

Mercury in the air and your risk of developing autism.

How close you live to a coal-fired power plant or other mercury-releasing industrial facility may affect your risk of developing autism.

In a landmark study from Texas, evaluation of data from the Texas Education Department and data from the United States Environmental Protection Agency showed a statistically significant association between autism risk and distance from the mercury source.

For every 1000 pounds of industrial release, there was a corresponding 2.6% increase in autism rates. When the mercury was associated with power plant emissions, there was a 3.7% increase in autism rates. The researchers found that community autism prevalence was reduced by 1 percent to 2 percent with each 10 miles of distance from the pollution source.[15]

Mitochondrial Dysfunction and Autism

Mitochondrial dysfunction is currently a major area of autism research.

Mitochondria - Mitochondria are one type of organelle inside the cell. Mitochondria produce energy. Mitochondria have their own genome, their own DNA. There is evidence that mitochondria originated from an ancient symbiosis between a nucleated cell and an oxygen-using non-nucleated cell. The mitochondria DNA resembles bacteria DNA. It is this similarity between mitochondria and bacteria that make the mitochondria susceptible to damage from many antibiotics.

A review was published in 2011, looking at four major areas of interest in autism research:
- immune dysregulation and inflammation
- oxidative stress
- mitochondrial dysfunction
- environmental toxicant exposures

Prior to 1986, only 12 publications were identified in the four major areas. However, in the time period of 2006 to 2010, there were 552 publications in these areas.

The authors found overlaps between these four major areas.

They found evidence that environmental toxicant exposures can induce immune dysregulation and/or inflammation, oxidative stress and mitochondrial dysfunction.[16]

Oxidative Stress - A disturbance in the balance between the production of reactive oxygen species (free radicals) and antioxidant molecules. Free radicals are produced during normal cellular functions. Free radicals cause damage within the cells.

Antioxidants neutralize free radicals. Antioxidants are produced by the body and also are found in foods.

Multiple Sensitivities and Autism

Why do children with autism have so many sensitivities?
Another model to help explain the interaction between a combination of factors is the **TILT, Toxicant-induced Loss of Tolerance**.[17] This model was built by Dr. Claudia Miller. Dr. Miller pulls together years of observation from numerous researchers in diverse fields of study. She has built a model to help explain the "loss of tolerance" that many people have developed to chemicals to which they were previously tolerant. Another term similar to "loss of tolerance" is "Multiple Chemical Sensitivity".

Illnesses associated with Multiple Chemical Sensitivity have been called by many names.
There is considerable overlap in the multitude of symptoms often seen in conjunction with Multiple Chemical Sensitivity.

Depending on the specific group of symptoms, the illnesses are called by many names, including (but not limited to):
- Fibromyalgia
- Chronic Fatigue Syndrome
- Gulf War Syndrome
- ADHD
- Autism
- Lupus
- IBS
- Reactive Airway Dysfunction Syndrome
- and many others

The organ systems affected include:
- Nervous System
- Cardiovascular
- Respiratory
- Gastrointestinal
- Connective tissue/Musculoskeletal
- Skin
- Airways of head (sinuses, ears, nose and throat)

Dr. Miller's model provides an explanation for, evidence for, a "reason" for the seemingly random, sudden, onset of what is sometimes an explosion of symptoms.

The TILT model may explain why a previously tolerated food becomes a significant trigger of symptoms.

With the TILT model, chemical sensitivity develops in two stages. The first stage is the loss of tolerance following acute or chronic exposure to various environmental agents (toxins).

The second stage is a triggering of symptoms by extremely small quantities of previously tolerated chemicals, drugs, foods, and food and drug combinations. This may explain why we see so many food sensitivities in a person who previously tolerated these foods. It may also explain why one person may not be affected by a medication or vaccine, yet another is. More information on the research of Dr. Claudia Miller can be found at http://drclaudiamiller.com/.

How does "TILT" relate to autism?

So part of our problem may be that all children are exposed in-utero (during pregnancy) to the mother's toxic burden. And then, depending on that child's toxic load and his or her ability to detoxify, a loss of tolerance to chemicals may develop. Part of the problem may also be, that some chemicals we are born with interfere with detoxification. This could contribute to the loss of tolerance to chemicals. Some of the chemicals we are born with also contribute to insulin resistance, but that is for another chapter.

Brain Injury, Encephalopathy, and Autism

What is the relationship between encephalopathy and autism?

Encephalopathy - a disease or disorder of the brain.

Children who had newborn encephalopathy were 5.9 times more likely than controls, to be diagnosed with an autism spectrum disorder.

Authors of a study published in 2006 were surprised to find that there was a strong association between newborn encephalopathy and autism spectrum disorders. By age 5 years, 5% of infants with newborn encephalopathy, and 0.8% of the controls were diagnosed with an autism spectrum disorder.

Compared with the controls, the children who had newborn encephalopathy were 5.9 times more likely to be diagnosed with an autism spectrum disorder.

The Inclusion criteria for children with moderate or severe newborn encephalopathy included: Either seizures alone or any two of the following lasting for longer than 24 hours - Abnormal consciousness; Difficulty maintaining respiration (of presumed central origin); Difficulty feeding (of presumed central origin); Abnormal tone and reflexes.

A relationship was demonstrated between newborn encephalopathy and autism, but how these two things are related to each other is still unclear.

The authors concluded that they were not sure about what their findings of the association between newborn encephalopathy and autism represented. Was this a case of common risk factors acting along independent pathways resulting in both the encephalopathy and autism? Or did these conditions share a common defect in fetal neurodevelopment? Another possibility they acknowledged, was that the encephalopathy itself either causes autism or is the first sign of underlying autism in a newborn infant. In this case, the infant encephalopathy and autism lie along the same causal pathway to neurological dysfunction.[18]

Is the term "chronic dynamic encephalopathy" a better description than "developmental disorder"?

Martha Herbert, MD, PhD, has actively studied children with autism for a number of years. She has been a forward-thinking leader in autism research. She suggests that we should consider using the term "chronic dynamic encephalopathy" instead of "developmental disorder". The chronic dynamic encephalopathy model encompasses the multiple neurological variations we see in children with autism. This model also is compatible with the variability in presentation we see within individuals and also is compatible with the idea of regression.

A changeable condition.

The term, chronic dynamic encephalopathy, implies that this condition is changeable, not static. She points out that many things we see associated with autism, that have been identified in neuropathology and imaging, may be caused by an underlying process, not a static cause of autism. These things include Purkinje cell loss or dysfunction that could be due to excitotoxicity; and white matter enlargement that could be due to inflammation.[19]

It may be toxins and inflammation causing changes we see in the brain, not a genetic mutation.

In other words, excitotoxicity (from toxins) and inflammation can cause changes that we see in the brain. And it is the toxins and the inflammation that are causing the changes in the brain that we see in autism, not a genetic mutation.

Dynamic (changeable), not hard-wired.

I think that it is very important for our model of the illness we call autism, to include an explanation for what parents see when their child regresses. In some cases, the regression was very sudden. In some cases, more gradual. And how do we explain those times when the autism fog seems to clear? Parents have described this phenomenon occurring when a child has fever or is on antibiotics. If autism were a static condition, this phenomenon could not occur.

Many parents have embarked on the Biomedical path and have seen significant improvement in their child. Again, this could not occur if autism were some hard-wired change in the circuits in the brain. There must be some explanation for the observed changes. A chronic dynamic encephalopathy is a good way to describe what we see.

The disease process that causes autism is actually a disease that affects the entire body.

Autism is a chronic condition, a chronic illness. Dynamic means that it changes. Encephalopathy means a disorder or disease of the brain. However, we are also learning that the disease processes that cause autism is actually more than a disease of the brain, it is a disease that affects the entire body.

Mother's Toxic Burden and Autism

To better understand our toxic burden, let's visit our tale of the orca whales again.

The Deep Blue Sea

People enjoy watching the orca whales of Puget Sound. Whale Watching has become a popular activity and people travel great distances to be able to watch these majestic animals in their native environment. Many of the whales have been named and families of whales are tracked and monitored. It brings us closer to the natural world when we watch these graceful creatures swim and interact. A casual observer might never guess what has been happening to these deep sea neighbors. Do *you* know what is happening to their babies?

What happens to the firstborn calf of an orca whale?
In many cases, the firstborn orca calf dies.

All of these orcas are contaminated with some amount of Polychlorinated Biphenyls (PCBs). PCBs, are members of a family of man-made chemicals called *chlorinated hydrocarbons*. The PCBs enter the water through spills, leaks, damage to equipment and improperly disposed trash.

The production of PCBs was banned in 1979 in the U.S. but the chemical is still in the environment.

PCBs are extremely fat-soluble, meaning they accumulate easily in fats. PCBs in the Puget Sound orcas come from their diet of Chinook salmon which have accumulated PCBs in their fat.

PCBs:
- lower orcas' immunity to diseases.
- decrease sperm count.
- disrupt many hormonal, developmental and reproductive processes.

Once in the orca, the toxins don't go away. These toxins build up in the fatty blubber of the orcas. As PCB concentration increases, it severely decreases the orca's lifespan.

Can any of the orcas decrease their level of PCBs?
Only sexually mature females have a chance of getting rid of any PCBs. While pregnant, some of the PCBs transfer to the developing offspring. After birth, even more toxins are transferred to the baby

when excreted through the mother's breast milk which is extremely rich in fat.

Having offspring increases the mother's chance of survival.

Studies show female blubber samples have one-third the levels of PCB toxins found in male orcas. Having offspring increases the mothers chance of survival.

However, the PCB levels in the developing calf, especially the first-born, often lead to its premature death.

It sometimes takes multiple attempts for female orcas to have a calf with low enough PCB levels to survive.[20] [21] [22]

Should we care about what is happening to the orcas?

Well, yes, I think we should. Actually, on many levels, we should care about what is happening to the orcas. As our deep sea neighbors, we should care about their health and well-being. As a reflection of what is happening to our own children, we should care about the tragedy unfolding. You see, chlorinated molecules such as PCBs are amazing things, and not in a good way. These are new, human-created molecules that may have appeared to solve other problems, but have wreaked havoc through multiple ecosystems and food webs, including our own. In the end, these and other modern chemicals have caused significant new problems.

The health crisis of the orcas gives us clues about our own current health crisis.

One of the items in our Venn diagram is Environmental Factors.

Environmental factors include the chemicals that we are exposed to as well as the food that we eat. Environmental factors include toxins.

When does exposure to toxins begin?

Toxin exposure does not begin after birth. Babies are born with a toxic burden. This means that before a baby is ever born, it is exposed to an unbelievable level of toxins that are circulating in the mother. This is not a problem limited to a few mothers. This is very likely happening to just about every mother in the world.

The Body Burden Study, commissioned by the Environmental Working Group (EWG), found up to **232 toxic chemicals** in the umbilical cord blood of 10 babies. These 10 children were born between December 2007 and June 2008 in Michigan, Florida, Massachusetts, California and Wisconsin.

What was found in the cord blood, in the blood circulating in the babies? There were 21 contaminants found for the first time in American newborns, including Bisphenol A (BPA). BPA is a synthetic estrogen that disrupts the endocrine system, disrupts normal reproductive system development and diminishes test animals' intellectual and behavioral capacity. According to the EWG, the chemicals found in these children are from unintended exposures to some of the most problematic consumer product and commercial chemicals ever put on the market. Besides the hormone disruptors, many of the chemicals are neurotoxins.

Ten of ten of the newborns had measurable levels of *lead, mercury, methylmercury and Polychlorinated biphenlys (PCBs).*

All of the chemicals found in the newborns had been part of the toxic body burden of the mother. While in the uterus, the mother's detoxification systems are helping to eliminate the toxins from her body and from the baby's body. Once born, the infant's liver now has the task of detoxifying chemicals all on its own.

What does the mother's toxic burden have to do with autism?

There are multiple studies and theories, pointing to different possible causes of this exploding epidemic of autism. In keeping with the current theme, I bring you this study from the University of Wisconsin-Madison. In the largest study of its kind, at the time of publication in 2008, researchers demonstrated that the risk of autism increases for firstborn children and children of older parents.

The study, led by epidemiologist Maureen Durkin, looked at more than 1,200 cases of autism. The research team looked at more than 200,000 U.S. births.

Higher risk for autism was seen in firstborn offspring of mothers who were older than 34 and fathers older than 29.

They found a 20% increase in the risk of autism with each 10-year increase in maternal age and a 30% increase in the risk of autism with each 10-year increase in paternal age. They also found that a couple's third or fourth child has significantly less risk than the first, regardless of the parents' ages.

The highest risk group included firstborn offspring of mothers aged >= 35 years and fathers aged >= 40 years, with a risk 3 times that of the reference group.

Part of the mother's toxic burden is transferred to her child during pregnancy.

One of the theories discussed included the firstborn's exposure to toxins. The chemicals a woman has acquired over her lifetime are either released directly into the fetus and/or passed through her breast milk.[23]

The firstborn child often has the greatest exposure to the mother's body burden of toxic chemicals.

Just as we saw with the orcas, the firstborn has the greatest exposure to the mother's body burden of toxic chemicals, and is often the most severely affected.

Where do these chemicals come from?

You might be amazed and appalled. Some of these are industrial chemicals, but many are chemicals that are found in many common, everyday things - pesticides in the foods we eat, chemicals in house-hold cleaning products, chemicals in pots and pans, and even chemi-cals found in cosmetics.

Can we change our body burden of toxins?

Unlike the orca, we can change our body burden of toxins. While we are still surrounded by many environmental toxins, what we eat and the products we use in our home can make a huge difference.

One of the very first things you can do, to help your child and to help yourself, is to begin to stop poisoning yourselves. We'll cover this more in a later chapter.

Pharmaceuticals and Autism

Is there a connection between the MMR vaccine and autism?

One of the major questions regarding pharmaceuticals, has been whether or not there is a connection between vaccines and autism. The vaccine that has had some of the most concern is the MMR vaccine.

Does the MMR vaccine cause autism?

There was a study published in the New England Journal of Medicine in 2002 that concluded that there was strong evidence against the hypothesis that MMR vaccination causes autism.[24] However, I think maybe we have been asking the wrong question.

When I look at the data from Table 2, which corrects for the num-ber of children who already had a diagnosis at the time of vaccination, the prevalence rate for autism disorder for unvaccinated children is

5.4 per 10,000. The prevalence rate for autism disorder for vaccinated children is 5.9 per 10,000. Is this statistically significant?

What if a more relevant question is, "Does the MMR vaccine contribute to an increase in autism prevalence in a population that is increasingly at risk due to other factors?" Other factors would include toxins associated with an increased risk for autism.

Another question should be, "What is in a vaccine that could be toxic?" The vaccine ingredients can be found on the package insert. One of the ingredients, that is found in the MMR vaccine, varicella (Chicken Pox) vaccine and the IPV (polio) vaccine, is Neomycin.[25]

What is Neomycin?
Neomycin is an aminoglycoside antibiotic. This type of antibiotic is toxic. Aminoglycoside antibiotics can be very toxic to the ear and kidneys of humans.

Neomycin is considered to be the most toxic of the aminoglycoside drugs.
High concentrations of neomycin in plasma (in the blood) can result in neomycin transfer to the fluid systems of the inner ear. The half-life in this fluid is 10 to 15 times longer than that in the blood stream. This means that compared to other parts of the body, the inner ear has a longer exposure time to the aminoglycoside drug.

Neomycin can be associated with nausea, vomiting, vertigo, nystagmus and difficulty with gait.
All aminoglycosides can affect both cochlear (hearing) and vestibular (balance) functions. However, with neomycin, it is hearing that is primarily affected. Perception of high-frequency sounds is lost first. Neomycin can cause vestibular toxicity with nausea, vomiting, vertigo, nystagmus and difficulty with gait.[26]

I could not find data on the lowest injected dose of Neomycin that was considered to be nontoxic.

The dose of neomycin in the vaccines is 25 mcg or less. Theoretically, this dose should be too low to be toxic. However, administration of neomycin parenterally (by injection into the muscle) is contraindicated due to its high toxicity to the ear and kidneys. I can't find data on the lowest parenteral (injected) dose that is considered to be nontoxic. This is probably because it is not to be given parenterally due to its toxicity.

The mechanism by which neomycin causes the damage appears to be a combination of:

    1. disruption of mitochondrial protein synthesis,

    2. the over-activation of NMDA glutamatergic receptors (N-methyl-D-aspartate),

    3. the formation of free radicals.

The disruption of mitochondrial protein synthesis occurs due to the similarity between mitochondrial DNA and bacterial DNA.

Neomycin enhances the function of the glutamatergic NMDA receptors because it mimics endogenous polyamines.[27]

All three of the mechanisms of neomycin damage have been connected to the damage we see in autism.

Endogenous - Part of self. Origin of the substance is within self.

Polyamines - A molecule that contains 2 or more amino groups. A protein is a molecule that is made up of multiple amino acids.

Please note that one of the toxic effects of neomycin is an over-activation of NMDA glutamate receptors. NMDA glutamate receptors are one area of study in both Autism research and Alzheimer's disease research.

Mitochondria are damaged by Neomycin.

An animal study looked at the microscopic damage caused by neomycin. Because damage first occurs in hair cells of the ear, they looked at hair cells on a zebrafish. These sensory cells are located externally on this fish. This makes these cells easy to observe.

When the animals were exposed to a low, 25 microMolar concentration of neomycin, the hair cells <u>had swollen mitochondria</u> but little other damage.

When treated with higher concentrations of neomycin, from 50 to 200 microMolar concentration, they had more severe cellular changes. The mitochondrial defects appear earlier and more predominantly than other cellular structural alterations.[28]

Neomycin is toxic to mitochondria.

Neomycin, given parenterally (by injection) can affect the flora in the gastrointestinal tract.[29]

Neomycin is noted to have the following possible effects:

"Neomycin is quickly and almost totally absorbed from body surfaces (except the urinary bladder) after local irrigation and when applied topically in association with surgical procedures. Delayed-onset irreversible deafness, renal failure and death due to neuromuscular blockade (regardless of the status of renal function) have been reported following irrigation of both small and large surgical fields with minute quantities of neomycin.

Cross-allergenicity among amino-glycosides has been demonstrated.

Aminoglycosides should be used with caution in patients with muscular disorders such as myasthenia gravis or parkinsonism since these drugs may aggravate muscle weakness because of their potential curare-like effect on the neuromuscular junction.

Small amounts of orally administered neomycin are absorbed through intact intestinal mucosa.

There have been many reports in the literature of nephrotoxicity and/or ototoxicity with oral use of neomycin. If renal insufficiency develops during oral therapy, consideration should be given to reducing the drug dosage or discontinuing therapy.

An oral neomycin dose of 12 grams per day produces a malabsorption syndrome for a variety of substances, including fat, nitrogen, cholesterol, carotene, glucose, xylose, lactose, sodium, calcium, cyanocobalamin and iron.

Orally administered neomycin increases fecal bile acid excretion and reduces intestinal lactase activity."[30]

NOTE: Cyanocobalamin is vitamin B12. Lactase is the enzyme that breaks down milk sugar.

Drugs.com lists the following *rare* side-effects for *oral* Neomycin:
loss of hearing
clumsiness
diarrhea
difficulty in breathing
dizziness
drowsiness
greatly decreased frequency of urination or amount of urine
increased amount of gas
increased thirst
light-colored, frothy, fatty-appearing stools
ringing or buzzing or a feeling of fullness in the ears
skin rash
unsteadiness
weakness[31]

Another toxin to avoid is acetaminophen.

Acetaminophen has been used as an over-the-counter medication in the United States since the 1960s. It is used to reduce fever and relieve pain. The most common brand of Acetaminophen is Tylenol.

Acetaminophen causes the depletion of glutathione.
Once in the body, the acetaminophen is converted to metabolic by-products which must then be cleared from the body. In the process of clearing the metabolic byproducts of acetaminophen, glutathione is used. Depending on the amount of acetaminophen being processed, glutathione can be significantly depleted.

Why do we need Glutathione?
Glutathione is an antioxidant. It is the major endogenous antioxidant produced in our cells. It can neutralize free radicals and can maintain vitamins C and E (these are also antioxidants) in their active forms.

Glutathione is used in many reactions in the cells. Every system in the body can be affected by the availability of active glutathione (reduced glutathione).

Reduced - a term used in chemistry that describes the "state" of a molecule. Glutathione in the *reduced form* acts as an antioxidant. Glutathione in the *oxidized form* does not function as an antioxidant. It must be regenerated into the "reduced" form to be usable again.

Glutathione can be depleted by acetaminophen. This can lead to a decrease in the availability of glutathione to act as an antioxidant. This can also lead to a decreased ability to detoxify toxic molecules.

When glutathione is completely depleted by acetaminophen, the toxic metabolite formed by acetaminophen destroys the liver cells.

This is the reason for avoiding toxic (lethal) doses of acetamino-phen. At sub-lethal doses, the ability of the body to detoxify and to neutralize free-radicals is compromised. At sub-lethal doses, the ability of the body to detoxify the ingredients of vaccines may be compromised.

Vaccines and your health.

To examine the risk and benefit of each vaccine is beyond the scope of this book. Vaccines are a medical procedure. All medical procedures have known risks. Many of the known risks (adverse reactions) will be printed on the package insert that can be provided for you to read. Anything listed as an adverse reaction has happened to someone. At the time of this writing, there is a website for the Immunization Action Coalition that has the inserts available on-line.

The website address is http://www.immunize.org/packageinserts/

Vitamin B12 Deficiency and Autism

Who needs vitamin B12?

I use a lot of vitamin B12 in my practice. One of the reasons for this, is that many of my patients have had GI tract disorders for a long time and have developed a deficiency of vitamin B12 (as well as some other nutrients). I also use vitamin B12 when there is evidence of neurological disease. Vitamin B12 is an essential nutrient for the maintenance and repair of the myelin covering around nerves.[32] I also treat with vitamin B12 when lab testing indicates a deficiency.

Most of the children I see in clinic will have a therapeutic trial of vitamin B12. Some have a very good response to the medication, some very little response.

Methylcobalamin, a form of vitamin B12, may be helpful in a subgroup of children.

There have been studies looking at the role of vitamin B12 in the treatment of autism.

In a pilot study published in 2010, there was no statistically significant mean difference in behavior tests or in glutathione status identified between the active and placebo groups.

However, in this study, 30% of the subjects demonstrated clinically significant improvement on the Clinical Global Impression

Scale and at least 2 additional behavioral measures. These responders exhibited significantly increased plasma concentrations of glutathione and the redox ratio of reduced glutathione to oxidized glutathione.

These findings suggests that the methylcobalamin (a form of vitamin B12) may alleviate symptoms of autism in a subgroup of children, possibly by reducing oxidative stress.[33]

Improvement was seen in a study using methylcobalamin and folinic acid.

In a study published in 2013, 37 children with autism were given methylcobalamin injections and folinic acid for 3 months. The Vineland Adaptive Behavior Scale (VABS) was utilized to monitor changes in behavior. Glutathione redox metabolites were measured at baseline and at the end of the 3 months.

All VABS subscales significantly improved. The authors noted that a greater improvement in glutathione redox status was associated with a greater improvement in expressive communication, personal and domestic daily living skills and interpersonal, play-leisure, and coping social skills. Treatment response was independent of age, gender and history of regression.[34]

Vitamin B6 and Autism

Vitamin B6 may be a very important nutrient when treating autism.

In 1978 an article appeared in the American Journal of Psychiatry. Sixteen autistic-type child outpatients had been identified who had appeared to have improved while taking vitamin B6. A double-blind study was done, with vitamin B6 and a matched placebo. Behavior was noted to have deteriorated during the vitamin B6 withdrawal.[35]

There may be a defect in the conversion of vitamin B6 to the active form.

Fast forward to 2006. An article was published showing that children with autism had abnormally high plasma levels of total vitamin B6 compared to controls. None of the children were receiving vitamin B6 supplements.

However, the active form of vitamin B6, pyridoxal 5' phosphate levels were low in the children with autism. These children appeared to have a low level of conversion of vitamin B6 to pyridoxal 5' phosphate.[36] This may explain why high doses of vitamin B6 have been found to be useful in children with autism.

If the conversion rate of a chemical is low, then by giving high doses of that chemical, the end result can be better levels of the active form.

While it is beyond the scope of this chapter, please be aware that it has been noted that Magnesium is an essential cofactor in many of the chemical pathways that utilize the active form of vitamin B6 (pyridoxal 5' phosphate).

Boys and Autism

Environmental toxins, toxic load, and endocrine disruptors may play a role in the higher ratio of boys to girls with autism.

To the best of my knowledge, no reason has been found for the higher ratio of boys to girls with a diagnosis of autism.

When we consider the possible role of environmental toxins, many of which are fat-soluble, I have a theory.

Let's talk about adults first. I see many adults with chronic conditions, such as fibromyalgia and chronic fatigue. In adults, there are more women with these conditions, than men. If fat-soluble toxins are playing a role, then the higher percentage of body fat that we see in women could contribute to their higher toxic load. Unlike the female orca that have multiple calves and decrease their toxic load, many women today have a limited number of children.

Using the data tables compiled by the WHO, I see that:

- for girls, the 50th percentile birth weight is 3.2322 kilograms.
- the 95th percentile birth weight is 4.040959 kilograms.
- for boys, the 50th percentile birth weight is 3.3464 kilograms.
- the 95th percentile birth weight of 4.214527.[37]

On average, boys weigh more than girls at birth. They would therefore, have a slightly higher toxic load at birth.

At 24 months, the 50th percentile weight for girls is 11.4775 kilograms.

For boys at 24 months, the 50th percentile weight is 12.1515 kilograms.

It would appear that boys would be taking on a greater toxic load, compared to girls, while breastfeeding.

Prenatal toxin exposure and increased risk for boys.

There is additional evidence, derived from studies looking at prenatal exposure to PCBs in rats, that the effects of the toxin on the developing male brain, are different from the effects on the developing female brain.[38]

One study looked at neurodevelopment, motor behavior, cerebellar structure, and protein expression in rat neonates exposed to the PCB mixture Aroclor 1254. The PCB exposure impaired performance on four behavioral tests, with the male pups more severely affected than female. Changes in behavior were associated with changes in cerebellar structure and protein expression.[39]

I wonder if the male pups weighed more than the female pups.

Chapter 4:

Risk Factors and Autism - Bridging the Gap Between Epidemiological Studies and Biochemistry

We have a lot of studies showing that a lot of different things are related to the risk of having autism. How do we bring all of this information together?

My goal, with this document, is to look at these various risk factors, find a common link, and determine how this common link can result in the symptoms, the set of behaviors, that we call autism. This common link should also help explain the "co-morbidities".

Many of us believe these "co-morbidities" are the actual "medical" and "biochemical" manifestations of the SYSTEMIC disease that results in the behaviors that we call autism.

One way of assessing information from multiple studies, is to use a meta-analysis.

Meta-analysis - "Meta-analysis is the use of statistical methods to combine results of individual studies. This allows us to make the best use of all the information we have gathered in our systematic review by increasing the power of the analysis. By statistically combining the results of similar studies we can improve the precision of our estimates of treatment effect, and assess whether treatment effects are similar in similar situations." (From: The Cochrane Collaboration open learning material.)[40]

A meta-analysis can also combine studies to look at risk factors for an illness.

In a study published in 2009, the authors provide a meta-analysis of the association between maternal pregnancy complications and pregnancy-related factors, and the risk of autism.

The factors with the strongest evidence for an association with autism risk included:

- advanced maternal and paternal age at birth
- maternal gestational bleeding
- gestational diabetes
- being first born vs third or later
- maternal prenatal medication use
- maternal birth abroad

However, in the analysis, the elevated risk of autism among the offspring of women born abroad was just shy of statistical significance.[41]

Maternal gestational diabetes was associated with a twofold risk of autism.

There was an 81% elevated risk associated with maternal bleeding during pregnancy. I suspect that it is the underlying cause of the bleeding that is related to the risk of autism.

Although an increased risk was seen with maternal medication use, the majority of the studies looked at the general use of any medication during pregnancy, not specific medications.

Thirteen studies were included in the meta-analysis of maternal age at birth. Maternal age at birth over 30 was associated with an increased risk. This risk ranged from a 27% increased risk (30 - 34 vs 25 - 29) to a 106% increase in risk (40+ vs < 30).

With their analysis of the data, they saw that for each 5-year increase in maternal age, there was an associated 7% increase in risk.

Increased paternal age at birth was also found to be significant, with a 5-year increase in paternal age associated with a 3.6% increase in risk. Four studies were included in the meta-analysis of paternal age. In three studies that examined the effect of young paternal age at birth, indicated a 26% decrease in risk for paternal age < 25.

The meta-analysis found a statistically significant 61% increase in risk for first-born children compared with children born third or later.

A further look at gestational diabetes and the risk of autism.

In a study published in the journal, Pediatrics, in 2012, the researchers looked at the relationship between:

- maternal metabolic conditions (diabetes, hypertension, and obesity),
- and the risk for autism and other neurodevelopmental disorders.

They found that diabetes, hypertension, and obesity were more common among mothers of children with autism spectrum disorders (ASD) and developmental disorders, compared to controls.

Diabetes was associated with statistically significantly greater deficits in expressive language among children with ASD. They note, at the end of the journal article, "The prevalence of obesity and diabetes among US women of childbearing age is 34% and 8.7%, respectively. Our findings raise concerns that these maternal conditions may be associated with neurodevelopmental problems in children and therefore could have serious public health implications."[42]

These studies show that we have evidence for the following significant risk factors:

1. Advanced maternal and paternal age at birth.
2. Maternal gestational bleeding.
3. Gestational diabetes.
4. Birth order (first more than fourth).
5. Maternal medication use during pregnancy.

Linking toxins, parental age, diabetes, medications and birth order.

We have other studies, noted elsewhere in the book, that show a link between toxins and autism. As we go through the next chapters, I will be showing you that at least 4 of the five items in the list above are connected to the toxic exposures. Maternal medications, are by definition, toxins.

Key links are mitochondrial dysfunction and insulin resistance.

Our key links are mitochondrial dysfunction and insulin resistance. We are going to see that toxins can lead to mitochondrial dysfunction, which can then lead to insulin resistance. The insulin resistance can lead to changes in brain function and behavior.

The toxins can also contribute to many of the comorbidities that we see, including impaired immune function and an increase in chemical sensitivity. The chemical sensitivity can be related to any molecule in food or the environment, even if previously tolerated, that can become a trigger for an immune reaction. Many of these toxins are also hormone disruptors or mimics, also contributing to comorbidities that we see in autism.

Do any of the factors related to an increased risk for autism also show a relationship with insulin resistance?

This is the question we are addressing next.

Chapter 5:

Autism and Insulin Resistance

Is there a relationship between autism and insulin resistance?
Previous chapters have looked at clues related to autism. Now, we are
going to shift our focus to looking at clues related to insulin resistance. Is it a coincidence that many of the factors we find associated
with autism are also associated with insulin resistance?

Let's look again at our Venn diagram.

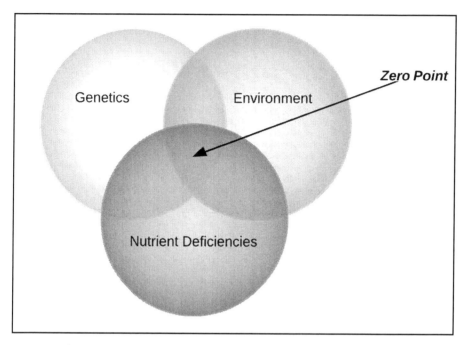

This Venn Diagram shows the overlap of GENETIC PREDISPOSITION, ENVIRONMENTAL FACTORS, and NUTRIENT DEFICIENCIES.

In the next chapter, we are going to take six of the factors associated with autism, and see how they are related to insulin resistance. Remember, these factors all are related to either/or:

- Genetics
- Environment
- Nutrient Deficiencies

Chapter 6:

Insulin Resistance Clues

Gluten and Insulin Resistance

Is there a relationship between gluten and insulin resistance?
I could not find many studies looking at gluten and insulin resistance.
I found one. A mouse study. But interesting.

Mice fed a gluten-free diet had less fat gain, less inflammation, and less insulin resistance.
One group of mice was fed a high-fat diet containing 4.5% Gluten (Control) and the other group had no gluten. **The Gluten-free mice had less fat gain, less inflammation, and less insulin resistance.** Since these were mice, it was assumed that the effects were independent of Celiac disease.[43]

Avoiding gluten may improve insulin resistance.
The results of this study suggests that avoiding gluten may improve insulin resistance, perhaps even in humans. If insulin resistance is related to autism, then this may be one mechanism whereby gluten avoidance is helpful.

It may be that many of the things that help with autism recovery are essentially helping to improve insulin sensitivity.

Let me repeat that.

It may be, that many of the things that help with autism recovery, are essentially helping to improve insulin sensitivity. Keep this statement in mind as we look for more clues in this chapter.

I consider gluten-containing foods to be "reactive" foods.

When a person is experiencing inflammation and symptoms, one of the first things we do is remove the most reactive foods, including gluten-containing foods. This does not fix the underlying problem, but can help to reduce inflammation and symptoms.

Heavy Metals, Air Pollution, Chlorinated Hydrocarbons, Herbicides, and Insulin Resistance

Is there any relationship between heavy metals and insulin resistance? Between air pollution and insulin resistance?

A study published in 2013 shows a link between long-term exposure to traffic-related air pollution and insulin resistance in children.

Insulin resistance increased by 17% for every 10.6 microgram/cubic meter increase in ambient nitrogen dioxide and 19% for every 6 microgram/cubic meter increase in particulate matter of up to 10 micrometer in diameter.

So the higher the exposure to traffic-related pollution, the greater this risk of developing insulin resistance.

Proximity to the nearest major road increased insulin resistance by 7% per 500 meters. All the findings were statistically significant.[44]

The closer you live to a major road, the greater your risk of developing insulin resistance.

In Chapter 3, in looking at the relationship between air pollution and autism, we learned that the combination of chlorinated chemicals and heavy metals is a dangerous duo.

Is the combination of chlorinated chemicals and heavy metals associated with an increase in insulin resistance?

A study from 2011 looked at the relationship between dioxins and mercury and an increased risk of insulin resistance.

Dioxins - a group of chlorinated hydrocarbons. One of the dioxins, TCDD, was an extremely toxic contaminant in Agent Orange. (PCBs are another group of chlorinated hydrocarbons.)

In this study, they found that insulin resistance increased with serum dioxins and blood mercury. Subjects with higher serum dioxins or blood mercury were at a significantly increasing risk for insulin resistance.

The simultaneous exposure to dioxins and mercury appears to heighten the risk of insulin resistance more than does individual exposure.[45]

So, again, the combination of chlorinated hydrocarbons and heavy metals, in this case mercury, is a more dangerous combination that either chemical group alone. We see that some of the things associated with autism are also associated with insulin resistance. Coincidence?

Chlorinated chemicals and diabetes.

And while we are on the topic of chlorinated hydrocarbons, let's take a look at PCBs and diabetes. Polychlorinated biphenyls (PCBs) manufactured in Anniston, Alabama, from 1929 to 1971 caused significant environmental contamination. The Anniston population remains one of the most highly exposed in the world.

The excess diabetes risk in females may be secondary to a higher percentage of body fat, allowing for a greater body burden of toxins.

Researchers recruited local volunteers to examine the relationship between body burden of PCBs and risk of diabetes. They observed significant associations between elevated PCB levels and diabetes, mostly in women and in individuals < 55 years of age. The authors note that the excess diabetes risk in exposed females may be secondary to a higher percentage of body fat, allowing for greater accumulation and retention of lipophilic (fat-soluble) compounds.[46]

A higher body burden of toxins puts females at greater risk of diabetes and also at greater risk of gestational diabetes. Do you remember what toxin is causing the loss of so many first-born orca whales?

Are these polychlorinated chemicals, such as dioxins, causing health problems anywhere else in the world?
Researchers in Japan, conducted a cross-sectional study with 1374 participants that were not occupationally exposed to dioxins and related compounds. These people were living throughout Japan during 2002 - 2006.

What was the body burden of toxins related to?
Their results suggest that body burden levels of dioxins and related compounds are associated with metabolic syndrome.

Metabolic syndrome was diagnosed when 3 or more of the following five criteria were met:
   a) body mass index >= 25.
   b) serum triglycerides >= 150.
   c) serum HDL < 40 mg/dL in men or < 50 mg/dL in women.
   d) systolic blood pressure >= 130 and/or diastolic blood pressure >= 85, or self-reported history of physician-diagnosed hypertension.
   e) HgA1C >= 5.6, or self-reported history of physician-diagnosed diabetes.

The dioxin-like polychlorinated biphenyls showed the highest association with metabolic syndrome. A high association was seen with PCB-126 and PCB-105. High blood pressure, elevated triglycerides and glucose intolerance were most closely associated with these pollutants.[47]

There is growing concern about childhood obesity and insulin resistance.

Childhood obesity and insulin resistance are recognized as a major health problem.[48]

Multiple chronic diseases are associated with insulin resistance including:

- Heart disease
- Type II Diabetes
- PCOS (polycystic ovarian syndrome)

A predisposition to certain cancers and to Alzheimer's disease is also now recognized.

Perhaps, the cause of childhood obesity and insulin resistance goes beyond sugar and a lack of exercise.

Some of the cause for this crisis has been attributed to the excessive sugars in the standard American diet, as well as a decline in physical activity. While there is much to be said for moving away from the standard American diet, towards a balanced diet of real foods, the reasons for the crisis in our youth and adults may go beyond the sugar and the lack of exercise.

Let's look at what may actually be a significant contributor to insulin resistance and obesity.

Could a common herbicide be linked to obesity?

In a study looking at a possible link between herbicide use and insulin resistance, scientists found an association between atrazine (ATZ, 2-chloro-4-ethylamine-6-isopropylamino-S-triazine) and obesity.[49]

The authors of this study note that this herbicide has been used in the United States since the early 1960s and that this time frame corresponds to the beginning of the obesity epidemic.

The map of AZT usage is very similar to the map of areas with higher concentrations of obesity in the United States.

In their study, a map of AZT usage shows that the "Corn Belt" region of the United States has the heaviest application. They also provide CDC data that shows a high concentration of individuals with a body mass index over 30 kg/m^2 in this area and the surrounding area with connected water sources.

AZT causes insulin resistance and obesity in rats.

The scientists found that chronic exposure to low concentrations of ATZ induced abdominal obesity and insulin resistance in rats by impairing mitochondrial function.

The use of AZT affected the structure and function of mitochondria.

Electron microscopy of the soleus muscle mitochondria showed that the mitochondria were swollen and their cristae were partially destroyed. They also found that AZT decreased the membrane potential of mitochondria and reduced intracellular ATP content in some cells.

AZT blocked the insulin-Akt signaling pathway.

Enzymatic activities of cytochrome bc_1 complex was decreased by 10% in the muscles of the AZT-treated animals. They also found that AZT treatment blocked the insulin-Akt signaling pathway. This may help explain the link between chronic AZT exposure and insulin resistance and weight gain.

This may also help explain the dramatic increase in other medical conditions, such as Alzheimer's disease, that is now being linked to insulin resistance.

Cytochrome bc1 - The third complex in the electron transport chain. This complex plays a role in the biochemical generation of ATP. ATP provides chemical energy within cells.

The link between AZT and corn-derived foods.

Several variations of a low-carbohydrate or lower-carb diet have become popular in the past few years. One of these, the "Paleo" diet, eliminates all grains from the diet. Perhaps, by eliminating grains, the followers of this style of eating are not only reducing their intake of carbohydrates and inflammatory grains, but are also reducing their intake of AZT and other agricultural toxins. If AZT is being introduced into humans through corn-derived foods, this may be a link between the fast food industry and obesity. The authors note that many products in a fast food restaurant are corn-derived, including the beef and chicken that are corn-fed.

Living in the "Corn Belt" may expose you to AZT through the water supply.

Those who live in the "Corn Belt" may be double challenged to reduce their AZT exposure. Not only would they need to decrease or eliminate their consumption of grains treated with AZT, they must find a source of pure water for drinking and cooking - water that is not contaminated with AZT.

Is there a link between mitochondrial dysfunction, insulin resistance and polychlorinated compounds?

There are some very interesting journal articles about mitochondrial dysfunction, insulin resistance and dioxin-like substances. I find these very interesting because there is a lot of evidence indicating a problem with mitochondrial dysfunction as a contributing factor in autism. And there is growing evidence indicating that insulin resistance may be a factor in autism. And then there is this link with dioxin-like substances when there is also evidence of toxins being a factor in the development of autism.

Mitochondrial DNA density in blood cells was lower in those who would go on to develop diabetes in 2 years, compared to those who would not.

This article, from the Diabetes and Metabolism Journal in Korea, looks at the link between mitochondrial dysfunction, insulin resistance and dioxin-like substances.[50] The author and colleagues had already noted, in previous studies, that blood mitochondrial DNA density in peripheral blood cells was lower in those subjects who would go on to develop diabetes in 2 years, in comparison to those who would not.

There is evidence that mitochondrial dysfunction may be the abnormality causing insulin resistance.

They later accumulated evidence suggesting that mitochondrial dysfunction might be the central abnormality causing insulin resistance. In the Sulwon Lecture of 2010, Professor Lee links insulin resistance with mitochondrial dysfunction.

Type 2 diabetes is a later stage of insulin resistance, not a separate disease.

Professor Lee also points out that type 2 diabetes is actually a later stage of insulin resistance, not a separate disease state. He presents an argument for insulin resistance to be a result of metabolic scaling law, that the body metabolism is changing in order to adapt to decreasing mitochondrial function. In other words, the state of insulin resistance is an adaptation of the body to the decrease in unit mitochondrial function.

What this means is that if you poison the mitochondria, and have less functional mitochondria, one way in which the body can adapt is by decreasing demand on the mitochondria. The way to decrease demand is to decrease response to insulin. So, if you poison your mitochondria, the way your body can adapt is to develop insulin resistance.

While this adaptation is a way for the organism to survive, if the loss of mitochondria is due to poisoning, the adaptation is not without consequences. For more information regarding this process, including a possible mechanism between type 2 diabetes and the development of coronary artery disease, I suggest you review this article yourself.

Professor Lee's three basic causes for type 2 diabetes: genes, developmental toxins, environmental toxins.

When looking at the many possible causes of type 2 diabetes, there have been many proposed models. In the mitochondria-based model, Professor Lee considers three basic causes: genes and developmental and environmental toxins.

Professor Lee considers the continuous accumulation of environmental toxins, the persistent organic pollutants (POPs) to be one of the most important factors.

"The most important cause of type 2 diabetes and the metabolic syndrome is environmental. Something bad was introduced during industrialization and is increasing in the environment." This something bad was not an infectious agent.

What are these persistent organic pollutants (POPs)?

POPs are defined as "chemical substances that persist in the environment, bio-accumulate through the food web, and pose a risk of causing adverse effects to human health and the environment" by the Stockholm Convention.

21 POPs were identified by the Stockholm Convention.

Pesticides: aldrin, chlordane, DDT, dieldrin, endrin, heptachlor, hexachlorobenzene, mirex, toxaphene, chlordecone, alpha hexachlorocyclohexane, beta hexachlorocyclohexane, lindane, pentachlorobenzene.

Industrial chemicals: hexachlorobenzene, polychlorinated bi-phenyls (PCBs), hexabromobiphenyl, hexabromodiphenyl ether and heptabromodiphenyl ether, pentachlorobenzene, perfluorooctane sulfonic acid, its salts and perfluorooctane sulfonyl fluoride, tetrabro-modiphenyl ether and pentabromodiphenyl ether.

Their byproducts are: hexachlorobenzene; polychlorinated diben-zo-p-dioxins and polychlorinated dipbenzofurans (PCDD/PCDF), and PCBs, alpha hexachlorocyclohexane, beta hexachlorocyclohexane and pentachlorobenzene.

I know, a lot of long, complicated-looking chemical names. But take another look at these chemical names. How many names do you see that contain one of the halogens (chloro-/chlorine, fluor-/fluorine, bromo-/bromine)?

Researchers have confirmed an association between serum POPs levels and type 2 diabetes and insulin resistance. Initial studies were done using NHANES 1999-2000 data. Further observations followed from many other countries.

Ingesting contaminated fish oil can contribute to insulin resistance in rats.

Professor Lee cited an animal study in which rats were given either a diet containing fish oil obtained from farmed Atlantic salmon, or fish oil that had been decontaminated with activated charcoal to remove POPs. The rats who ingested the crude (not decontami-nated) fish oil developed insulin resistance, abdominal obesity and fatty liver.[51]

Professor Lee makes what I consider to be a very important ob-servation. That only *certain* high-fat diets cause obesity in susceptible animals and that this high-fat diet was found to be contaminated with POPs. So, there is a very strong possibility that it is the poisons, the POPs, causing the obesity, not the actual fat in the diet.

Can we reverse the insulin resistance?

The mitochondria-model of insulin resistance suggests that if we can improve mitochondrial function, insulin resistance might decrease. To do this, we need to remove POPs and repair mitochondria.

Brain Injury, Encephalopathy and Insulin Resistance

In Chapter 3, we saw an association with encephalopathy and autism. Is there an association between encephalopathy and insulin resistance?

According to Dr. Sima of Wayne State University, diabetic encephalopathies are now accepted complications of diabetes.[52]

The underlying mechanisms leading to the cognitive deficits differs in type 1 and type 2 diabetes, but the encephalopathy occurs in both types of diabetes.

The increased incidence of Alzheimer's disease in type 2 diabetes appears to be associated with insulin resistance and the associated co-morbidities.

The type 1 diabetic encephalopathy involves learning abilities, intelligence development and memory retrieval. The underlying insulin deficiency has effects on the expression of neurotrophic factors, neurotransmitters, oxidative and apoptotic stressors. This results in defects in neuronal integrity and connectivity in the developing brain.

Insulin resistance and/or a lack of insulin can result in encephalopathy.

Dr. Sima discusses the effects of insulin and IGF-1 (insulin-like growth factor 1) in the brain. Not only in glucose utilization and energy metabolism, but also oxidative stress and gene regulation.

He also discusses Type 1 DM and children, pointing out that early onset of Type 1 DM results in worse neuropsychological performances and that males are more vulnerable than females. The pathophysiology in Type 1 DM includes an increase in oxidative stress.

Another observation I would like to make about diabetes, is that not all cases are clearly either Type 1 or Type 2, but there are some cases that appear to be a mix of the two types. Also, it is becoming more recognized that Type 2 DM is actually a part of the "disease" or "condition" of Insulin Resistance. In other words, Type 2 DM is what occurs when the Insulin Resistance progresses to the point that the blood glucose is elevated.

It is the Insulin Resistance that is the "disease", but the root of the Insulin Resistance appears to be the Mitochondrial Dysfunction.

The Mitochondrial Dysfunction may be due to poisoning, as indicated in an earlier chapter.

Insulin Resistance and Mitochondrial Dysfunction
We learned in Chapter 3 that much of the current research in autism is looking at mitochondrial dysfunction.

Is there a relationship between insulin resistance and mitochondrial dysfunction?
As I have mentioned, there is an increasing body of evidence linking mitochondrial dysfunction and insulin resistance. I'll give you examples of two more studies here.

Mitochondrial dysfunction occurs before there is evidence of insulin resistance.
One is a rat study, looking at the temporal (time) relationship between the development of mitochondrial dysfunction, "fatty liver", and insulin resistance. Fatty liver, now called nonalcoholic fatty liver disease (NAFLD), affects about 30% of all US adults and 75 to 100% of obese individuals. NAFLD is now considered the liver complication of metabolic syndrome (from insulin resistance).

The study group was a sedentary, hyperphagic obese, strain of rats. The control group was non-hyperphagic.

At 5 weeks of age, the study group was compared to the control group of rats. Serum insulin and glucose were the same between groups. However, the study animals had significant liver mitochondrial dysfunction. This was measured by looking at liver carnitine palmitoyl-CoA transferase-1 activity, fatty acid oxidation and cytochrome c protein content, compared to controls.

By 8 weeks, liver trigyceride levels were elevated in the study group, and by 13 weeks, insulin resistance had developed in the study group.[53]

So, by the time insulin resistance is evident, mitochondrial dysfunction is already present. It appears that it is the mitochondrial dysfunction that comes first, not the other way around.

Severity of insulin resistance correlated with the extent of mitochondrial dysfunction.

A study published in 2013 looked at adipocytes. Adipocytes are simply fat cells, cells that store fat.

In this study, the scientists induced mitochondrial dysfunction and overproduction of reactive oxygen species (ROS). An excess of reactive oxygen species is called "Oxidative Stress".

With these cells that had an increase in "Oxidative Stress", the researchers found a decrease of the insulin response as indicated by lower glucose uptake and decreased phosphorylation of Akt upon insulin stimulation. Also, the expression of glucose transporter 4 (Glut4) was decreased (this means, that the mechanism for moving glucose into the cell (Glut4) was decreased).

They also noted that the severity of insulin insensitivity (insulin resistance) was correlated with the extent of mitochondrial dysfunction.[54] In other words, the more severely the mitochondria were poisoned, the more severe the insulin resistance.

For years, we have blamed the patient for his or her disease.
I'd like to bring your attention to a very important point. You may
have realized this already as you have read this material on mitochondrial dysfunction and insulin resistance, as well as a preceding section
on toxic chemicals and insulin resistance.

For years, we in the medical field have blamed the patient for
his or her disease. We have blamed the patient with Type 2 DM for
being obese and developing diabetes. We have blamed the patient
for not being able to control his or her disease with diet and exercise. And we have blamed the patient when the disease progressed.
I think it is time that we recognize that we have been blaming the
wrong person.

Type 2 DM is an end product of Insulin Resistance. Insulin
Resistance is an end product of mitochondrial dysfunction.
Mitochondrial dysfunction, in the majority of cases, is due to poisoning of the mitochondria. Therefore, people with Type 2 DM have been
poisoned. It is not their fault.

Now, this does not mean that regulation of insulin and blood
sugar cannot be improved with diet. It can. A low carbohydrate
diet, based on real food, can play a key role in maintaining blood
sugar within the normal range. However, even with this diet, the
Insulin Resistance is still present, because the mitochondria are still
damaged.

**To reverse Insulin Resistance, we must stop poisoning our-
selves and we must take measures to restore mitochondrial
health.**
To truly reverse the Insulin Resistance, we must stop poisoning
ourselves.

To truly reverse the Insulin Resistance, it takes more than diet and
exercise.

To truly reverse the Insulin resistance, we must take measures to restore mitochondrial health.

Sheep that were deficient in vitamin B12 had abnormalities within the mitochondria.

One of the nutrients related to mitochondrial health is vitamin B12. A study of vitamin B12-deficient sheep found that the mitochondria in the muscle appeared to have been affected. Electron microscopy revealed abnormalities within the mitochondria structure.[55]

Could there also be a relationship between vitamin B12 deficiency and insulin resistance?

Let's go to the next section to find out.

Vitamin B12 Deficiency and Insulin Resistance

Maternal vitamin B12 deficiency was associated with an elevated risk of insulin resistance.

A group of almost 5000 pregnant women and their offspring were studied in Nepal. Maternal vitamin B-12 deficiency was associated with an elevated risk of insulin resistance. Of the women who were deficient in vitamin B12 in early pregnancy, their children had a 26.7% increase in HOMA-IR (an insulin resistance score).[56]

HOMA-IR - Homeostasis model assessment of insulin resistance. This is calculated using the level of fasting glucose and the fasting insulin.

Children of mothers with both high folate and low vitamin B12 were the MOST insulin resistant.

Another study looking at vitamin B-12 and folate status in pregnancy, also showed an association with maternal vitamin B12 deficiency and risk of insulin resistance. However, the children of mothers with a combination of high folate and low vitamin B12 concentrations were the most insulin resistant.[57]

Clinical finding - a high folate level may actually indicate a need for folate.

One thing I have noted in clinic, is that a high folate level may actually correspond to a need for folate in some cases. One of the clues we look for in the lab testing is the Formiminoglutamic acid (FIGlu) level. This is part of the urine testing that we do.

The increase in serum folate results from the severity of the vitamin B12 deficiency.

One possible explanation for this is that the increase in serum folate results from the severity of the vitamin B12 deficiency.

In the body, folate monoglutamates are elongated to polyglutamates within the tissue. However, 5-methyl-tetrahydrofolate cannot be easily elongated by folate polyglutamate synthase. In other words, the 5-methyl-tetrahydrofolate must first be altered. It must be demethylated to tetrahydrofolate (in a vitamin B12-dependent reaction) before being polyglutamated.

Vitamin B12 is necessary for changing the 5-methyl-tetrahydrofolate to tetrahydrofolate.

In severe vitamin B12 deficiency, the 5-methyl-tetrahydrofolate cannot be efficiently demethylated to tetrahydrofolate. Therefore, it cannot be polyglutamated or retained by the cell. This is the "methyl-trap" hypothesis.

The consequence of this is that the serum-tissue concentration gradient collapses and serum folate is no longer efficiently taken up by the tissue. The concentration of folate increases in the serum. The concentration of the tissue folate, particularly the more biologically active polyglutamates, decrease.[58]

When you supplement with 5-methyl-tetrahydrofolate, you must ensure that there is adequate vitamin B12 available.
This is one of the reasons, that when you supplement with an active form of folate, you must ensure that there is adequate vitamin B12 available.

Concentrations of vitamin B12 were lower in PCOS patients with insulin resistance compared to PCOS patients without insulin resistance.
We can also see a link between vitamin B12 deficiency and insulin resistance in other populations.

Patients with polycystic ovary syndrome (PCOS) were compared to a control population matched by age and body mass index. The relationship between vitamin B12 and insulin resistance was examined.

In PCOS patients, homocysteine concentrations and HOMA-IR (a measure of insulin resistance) were higher. Concentrations of vitamin B12 were lower in PCOS patients with insulin resistance compared to PCOS patients without insulin resistance. The vitamin B12 concentrations were significantly lower in obese PCOS women in comparison with obese control women.

Overall, insulin resistance, obesity and elevated homocysteine were associated with lower serum vitamin B12 concentrations in PCOS patients.[59] Note: Homocysteine is often elevated with vitamin B12 deficiency and/or folate deficiency.

Folic acid and vitamin B12 can reduce insulin resistance.
In a group with metabolic syndrome, the addition of folic acid and vitamin B12 for one month resulted in a significant reduction in insulin, insulin resistance, endothelial dysfunction and homocysteine levels.[60]

These studies, demonstrating of a link between vitamin B12 deficiency and insulin resistance, are a clue that there may be

a link between insulin resistance and other conditions that respond to vitamin B12 replacement.

Vitamin B6 and Insulin Resistance

Vitamin B6 has been shown to improve blood glucose levels in gestational diabetes.

As we saw in Chapter 3, children with autism appear to have a slower conversion rate of vitamin B6 to the active form, pyridoxal 5' phosphate. Or, it may be an imbalance between this conversion rate, and the rate of degradation (breaking down) of the active form. This could have an impact on any or all of the over 100 chemical pathways that utilize vitamin B6.

The oldest study I found looking at vitamin B6 and autism was published in 1978. If we go back to 1977, we can find vitamin B6 improving blood glucose levels in gestational diabetes. The findings of this study suggested that a relative deficiency in vitamin B6 was associated with some cases of gestational diabetes and that the replacement of this vitamin improved the insulin resistance.[61]

Do women who develop gestational diabetes have a deficiency of vitamin B6?

When we look at the top statistical risks for having a child with autism, what do we find? According to our list in Chapter 3, one of the risks is maternal gestational diabetes.

Could it be that women who develop gestational diabetes have a deficiency of the active form of vitamin B6, pyridoxal 5' phosphate? Could this deficiency be secondary to liver impairment due to toxins?

In severe liver disease, it may be an increased rate of destruction of the active form of vitamin B6 that leads to the deficiency.

There is evidence that in patients with severe liver disease, it may be an increased rate of degradation of pyridoxal 5' phosphate (the active form of vitamin B6) that leads to the vitamin B6 deficiency.[62]

Is it the lack of vitamin B6 that is the link between gestational diabetes and autism?

Vitamin B6 deficiency is associated with many illnesses, including the formation of kidney stones.

An interesting study looked at the effects of vitamin B6 on the livers of diabetic rats. Sometimes, when reading a study, you come across some additional interesting information.

In their introduction, the study authors note the importance of vitamin B6 regarding the number of chemical reactions that it participates in.

Then, they give an interesting list of conditions that vitamin B6 deficiency has been associated with (with references).

This list includes:

1. fatty liver
2. low insulin-like activity in the serum and pancreas
3. accumulation of total lipids (mainly of triglycerides and cholesterol ester in liver)
4. formation of calcium oxalate stones in the kidney
5. reduction of glycogen, glucose and alanine in the liver
6. carcinogenesis (developing cancer)
7. premature (young age) ischaemic (lack of oxygen) heart disease
8. immunological decline observed in persons infected with HIV

They also noted the effectiveness of vitamin B6 for:

1. heme synthesis (heme is in hemoglobin, in red blood cells)
2. hyperprolactinemia (elevated levels of prolactin, a hormone that promotes milk production) that can cause galactorea-amenorrhea (galactorea - producing milk) (amenorrhea - absence of menstrual period)
3. nausea due to pregnancy and radiotherapy (radiation treatment)
4. retinopathy (disease of retina of the eye)
5. gestational diabetes
6. nephropathy (kidney disease) and vascular diseases (diseases associated with arteries and veins)

In their study, they used streptozotocin (STZ) to induce diabetes in rats. STZ is toxic to pancreatic beta cells (beta cells are the cells that produce insulin).

There were 4 groups of rats.

1. Group I, controls
2. Group II, controls that received vitamin B6
3. Group III, STZ-treated (diabetic) rats
4. Group IV, STZ-treated (diabetic) rats that received vitamin B6

Vitamin B6 reduced liver damage in the diabetic rats.

When the livers of the animals were examined:

- both groups of control animals had liver tissue that was similar in appearance.
- the Group III rats (diabetic) showed liver damage.
- the Group IV rats (diabetic with vitamin B6) showed minimal liver damage.

The blood glucose level was significantly elevated (about 3 times higher) than baseline in the STZ rats.

The STZ + Vitamin B6 rats had elevated blood glucose, but about 2 times higher than baseline.

A similar pattern was seen in the liver enzymes, with the STZ rats having a significant elevation and the STZ + Vitamin B6 rats having less of an elevation.

Another measured parameter was the body weight of the rats. The loss of body weight in STZ-induced diabetes is due to the increased muscular wasting that we see in diabetes.

The STZ + Vitamin B6 rats, had about half the weight loss as the STZ only rats.[63]

Vitamin B6 is a coenzyme that works with AST and ALT.

The liver enzymes, aspartate transaminase (AST) and alanine transaminase (ALT), are seen in increased levels in the blood, when there is liver damage from disease or toxins. The activity of these enzymes is affected by availability of vitamin B6. Vitamin B6 is a coenzyme ("works with an enzyme") that works with AST and ALT.

Their study showed, that not only did the vitamin B6 protect the liver from damage in the STZ-induced diabetes, it also helped to improve the blood glucose level and decrease the weight loss that is seen in diabetes. Since the weight loss is due to loss of muscle mass, it is possible that the vitamin B6 is helping to preserve the health of mitochondria.

If vitamin B6 reduces loss of muscle mass in diabetes, is it actually helping to preserve the health of the mitochondria?

Chapter 7:

Autism, Alzheimer's Disease and Insulin Resistance

Is there a connection between Autism and Alzheimer's Disease?

So, now we get to the heart of the matter. How do you have a young child with neurotypical behavior one day, then in a matter of hours or days, begin to have aggression, and/or loss of speech, and/or loss of eye contact, and/or screaming, and/or....?

It may be that the process that is occurring at the cellular level in Alzheimer's Disease is similar to the process that is occurring at the cellular level in Autism. And there is accumulating evidence that insulin and Insulin Resistance play a role.

What happens when there is Insulin Resistance?

With Insulin Resistance, it requires more and more insulin to get the cell to respond to glucose, or to get glucose within the cell to be used for energy production. An elevated level of insulin, affects the cell in additional ways, including having an effect on glutamate receptors.

Some parts of the brain are more dependent on insulin than others.

It appears that there are some parts of the brain that are more dependent on insulin than others. With inadequate insulin signaling, there is inadequate glucose utilization in these areas of the brain, leading to changes in focus, comprehension, and speech.

The areas of the brain that perform the higher levels of functioning are not working well. The areas of the brain that have been associated with basic survival are functioning even with lower response to insulin.

This is illustrated in a study of basal insulin (*the baseline level of insulin, the minimal amount of insulin always circulating in the body*) and regional brain glucose uptake.

They found that the basal insulin has a role in regulating brain glucose, mostly in the cortical (*the gray matter*) areas of the brain. It is the cortex that plays a major role in:

- memory
- attention
- perceptual awareness
- thought
- language
- consciousness

When the circulating insulin fell below the basal level, there was a reduction in brain glucose uptake. There is, however, also *insulin-independent* brain glucose uptake. Overall, the brain will continue to take up glucose even with a decrease in basal insulin.

The areas that are sensitive to the decrease in insulin, the cortical areas, may not function as well when there is insufficient insulin, but the *areas of the brain critical to immediate survival*, i.e., the brain stem and cerebellum, *will continue to function.*[64]

Low insulin stimulation and behaviors.

Can you see how this might affect behavior? If the cortex is not functioning, the ability to pay attention and interact with another can be affected. Memory function is compromised, as is language.

The behaviors you might see would include anxiety, fear, running, screaming, and aggressive behaviors. These behaviors can be seen in people with autism and these behaviors can be seen in people with Alzheimer's disease.

Insulin treatment for Alzheimer's disease?

There is currently a clinical trial recruiting patients with Alzheimer's disease. This trial will study the effects of intranasally-administered insulin on cognition, memory and daily function, and also look at cerebrospinal fluid biomarkers.[65]

While this does not treat the root cause, this study can give us more clues about the biochemical changes occurring and the possible role of insulin in both the cause and treatment of this disease.

A previous study had looked at 2 different doses of intranasally-administered insulin compared to placebo. This study demonstrated;
- improved delayed memory
- preserved caregiver-rated functional ability.

Both insulin doses also preserved general cognition. Patients who received placebo showed decreased glucose uptake in several cortical regions, including parietotemporal and frontal regions. No treatment-related severe adverse events occurred during this trial.[66]

Higher Insulin Resistance is related to a decrease in gray matter and also to medial temporal lobe atrophy.

A study using an assessment of insulin resistance, HOMA-IR, looked at the role of Insulin Resistance in Alzheimer's disease.

HOMA-IR - Homeostasis model assessment of insulin resistance. This is calculated using the level of fasting glucose and the fasting insulin.

Higher Insulin Resistance was related to less gray matter at baseline (the beginning of the study) and 4 years later. The gray matter was less in the medial temporal lobe and prefrontal cortex. The higher Insulin Resistance was related to medial temporal lobe atrophy. This atrophy corresponded to cognitive deficits (problems with learning) in the Auditory Verbal Learning Test that was used during the study.[67]

Temporal Lobe - Plays a role in:
- memory
- processing sensory input
- comprehending language
- emotion

The temporal lobe contains the hippocampus.

Brain Insulin Resistance may occur independently of diabetes.

Brain Insulin Resistance has been shown to occur in patients without diabetes. The hippocampal formation and the cerebellar cortex in people with Alzheimer's disease were shown to have a reduced response to insulin signaling. There was a reduced response to insulin signaling in the insulin receptor to PI3K signaling pathway. There was also a reduced responses to Insulin-like Growth Factor 1 (IGF-1), in the IGF-1 to PI3K signaling pathway. The level of reduced response corresponded to the level of cognitive impairment.[68]

Their findings show both Insulin Resistance and resistance to IGF-1 in the brain of people with Alzheimer's disease. This can occur in the absence of diabetes.

Another interesting finding in this same study, was that Nitrotyrosine, a marker of inflammatory and oxidative stress associated with insulin resistance in Type 2 Diabetes, was elevated in Alzheimer's Disease cases.

In searching for the cause of the Insulin Resistance in the brain, they looked at insulin receptor activation and insulin-induced signaling molecules. The major reduction in insulin-induced signaling occurred "downstream" from the insulin receptor itself. These reductions were significant in the hippocampal formation.

They also note that insulin plays many roles in the brain, including formation and placement of NMDA and $GABA_A$ receptors.

The authors favor the term *insulin-resistant brain state* over the proposed term of Type 3 diabetes. Their reasoning is, that the insulin resistance they found in Alzheimer's Disease brains was not associated with elevated glucose levels.

Both Brain Insulin Resistance and Insulin Deficiency are related to Alzheimer's Disease.

An excellent article reviewing the evidence regarding insulin and Alzheimer's Disease, was written by Suzanne M. de la Monte. She cites evidence that the deficits in insulin and IGF (insulin-like growth factor) signaling are due to the combined effects of:

1. insulin and IGF resistance
2. deficiency of insulin

Because there is evidence of both insulin resistance AND insulin deficiency, she has proposed that Alzheimer's Disease be referred to as "Type 3 diabetes".[69]

What does all this information about Insulin Resistance mean?

I have been showing you the evidence that shows a relationship between:

- Insulin Resistance and Alzheimer's Disease.
- Areas of the brain affected by the Insulin Resistance and Alzheimer's Disease correspond to some of the symptoms we see in Autism.
- Insulin Resistance and Autism.
- Exposure to toxins such as POPs, including polychlorinated compounds, and Autism.

- Exposures to toxins such as heavy metals, including mercury, and Autism.
- Exposures to toxins such as POPs, including polychlorinated compounds, and Insulin Resistance.
- Exposures to toxins such as heavy metals, including mercury, and Insulin Resistance.
- Vitamin B6 deficiency and Autism.
- Vitamin B6 deficiency and Insulin Resistance.
- Mitochondrial dysfunction and Toxins.
- Mitochondrial dysfunction and Insulin Resistance.
- Mitochondrial dysfunction and Autism.
- Gluten sensitivity and Autism.
- Gluten exposure and Insulin Resistance.
- Vitamin B12 deficiency and Autism.
- Vitamin B12 deficiency and Insulin Resistance.
- Neomycin and Mitochondrial damage.
- Neomycin is a component of MMR vaccine, Varicella vaccine and the injected Polio vaccine.
- Depleted Glutathione and compromised ability to clear toxins.
- Depletion of Glutathione by Acetaminophen.

I have also been showing you evidence of decreased cortical function (decreased brain function) with either insufficient insulin, and/or insufficient response to insulin (Insulin Resistance), even when glucose levels are not elevated.

I look for patterns. And connections. What do you see when you look at this list?

This is what I see:

Genetics: Decreased detoxification capacity.

Environment: More toxins that the person has the capacity to detoxify.

These toxins then contribute to Mitochondrial Dysfunction which then results in Insulin Resistance.

Nutrient Deficiencies (B6, B12, Iodine [Chapter 10]) contributing to Insulin Resistance.

The **Zero Point** - Insulin Resistance at the root of:

Autism

Alzheimer's Disease

Heart Disease

Diabetes (type 2)

Degenerative Diseases

Many types of Cancer

How would you repair this broken system?

Would you look for a drug to treat the insulin resistance, or, would you want to repair the mitochondria and regain normal cellular function?

I vote for mitochondrial repair. This means we are going to have to do something about all the poisons and also, replace needed nutrients.

Chapter 8:

What about Secretin?

Secretin was a clue!

In 1996, a little boy named Parker Beck was seen by a gastrointestinal specialist. Parker had chronic diarrhea and the doctor was looking for evidence of celiac disease and also did a secretin challenge test. Soon after testing, Parker's bowel movements normalized and his parents saw dramatic improvement in his behavior. They reported improved speech, better eye contact and he was more social.

No reason could be found for his improvement. There was no known connection between the testing done and his improvements.

Parker's mother, Victoria Beck contacted many researchers but there was little interest in secretin. However, Dr Bernard Rimland, a founder of the Autism Research Institute (ARI), was very interested. Researchers associated with ARI began trying to figure out how the secretin could be working.

Research studies began. Phase I and Phase II studies were completed.

A company called Repligen purchased the patent rights for the use of secretin in the treatment of autism. Parker had been treated with porcine (pig) secretin, but Repligen developed a synthetic form. Research studies for FDA approval began.

Phase 1 studies were done to check for adverse reactions. Very few adverse effects were reported and secretin went on to Phase 2. For Phase 2, studies were conducted at 5 autism centers and involved 126 individuals with autism. All subjects had to have at least one GI problem. Phase 2 results were considered impressive and secretin went on to Phase 3 studies.

The subset of subjects with high-functioning autism showed a significant improvement.

In the Phase 3 studies, only 30% of the participants suffered from GI problems. When the double-blind code was broken, there was no difference seen between the test groups. However, when the data was further analyzed, the subset of subjects with high-functioning autism showed a significant improvement. The subset of subjects that improved dramatically, involved slightly more than half of the participants in the study.

According to research from ARI, secretin has been found in at least 3 areas of the brain (as well as the GI tract), including the hippocampus, the amygdala, and the cerebellum.

The Autism Research Institute conducted surveys that showed Secretin had very positive ratings by the parents.

For more than 30 years, ARI surveyed parents about their children's response to various treatments. Secretin had very positive ratings. Of 468 individuals, 44% responded positively to a secretin infusion. Of 196 individuals, 37% responded positively to a transdermal application of secretin. Negative ratings (children scored as worse after secretin treatment) were 7% and 10% respectively.[70]

What does secretin do?

So what does secretin do? Secretin stimulates the release of pancreatic secretions, such as bicarbonate, that aid digestion and help regulate acid/base balance in the small intestine. So, how does this help in autism?

It may be that the secretin helps with the chronic diarrhea and the acid/base balance. But, this would not necessarily explain the other changes seen - the improved behavior, improved speech, better eye contact and more social behavior. I am not denying the gut-brain connection. But, could there be something else that secretin is doing?

Surprise! Secretin is the GI stimulus for insulin release!

Secretin is the gastrointestinal stimulus for insulin release.[71] In a study with 3 different patterns of intravenous (IV) infusion of secretin, the integrated changes in insulin levels through the total infusion period were related to the total doses of secretin. With each dose of secretin, glucose tolerance was improved.[72]

I think that it is widely recognized that all people with autism do not have exactly the same broken physiology, the same broken biochemistry. This is a systemic illness arising from a combination of toxins, compromised ability to detoxify, and a changing demand for glucose and insulin in the brain.

It may be, that the subset of individuals in the secretin study who responded well to the secretin, were individuals who could respond well to additional insulin. We don't know the toxic level of the individuals in the study, but my guess is, that the "high functioning" individuals were relatively less toxic than the others and could therefore respond to the additional insulin released as a result of the secretin infusion.

Which is support for my recommendation to first "Stop Poisoning Yourself!" You cannot even begin to detoxify if you continue to poison yourself. We'll cover this more in a future chapter.

To get the poisons out, you must first stop putting them in!

Chapter 9:

Polychlorinated Biphenyls

A mother with gestational diabetes may have a greater toxic load due to having an increased amount of body fat which stores the fat-soluble toxins.

The older a mother is when pregnant with her first child, the greater her body burden of toxins, including PCBs. With each pregnancy, her body burden decreases, therefore, each subsequent child receives a smaller toxic load. The exception would be when there is a gap of a number of years between pregnancies, allowing time for accumulation of toxins.

A mother with gestational diabetes has insulin resistance. Is the greater risk for a child from autism due directly to the insulin resistance of the mother, and possibly an epigenetic switch flip? Or is the greater risk because the mother has a greater toxic load that is contributing to or causing the insulin resistance? A mother with gestational diabetes may have a greater toxic load due to having an increased amount of body fat which stores the fat-soluble toxins.

Let's look at what we know about PCBs.

PCBs are chlorinated hydrocarbons.

Polychlorinated Biphenyls, PCBs, are members of a family of man-made chemicals called *chlorinated hydrocarbons*.

Chlorinated hydrocarbon - An organic compound (contains carbon) that contains at least one bonded atom of chlorine.

PCPs were banned but have not disappeared.

PCBs were produced from 1929 to 1979. Although the production of PCBs was banned in 1979, these chemicals persist in the environment and in the food web. The PCBs are also still present in equipment that was manufactured before the ban.

PCBs have a range of toxicity. They were used in hundreds of industrial and commercial applications including electrical, heat transfer, and hydraulic equipment; as plasticizers in paints, plastics and rubber products; in pigments, dyes and carbonless copy paper; and many other industrial applications.

Products that may contain PCBs include:

- transformers and capacitors
- other electrical equipment including voltage regulators, switches, reclosers, bushings, and electromagnets
- oil used in motors and hydraulic systems
- old electrical devices or appliances containing PCB capacitors
- fluorescent light ballasts
- cable insulation
- thermal insulation material including fiberglass, felt, foam, and cork
- adhesives and tapes
- oil-based paint
- caulking
- plastics
- carbonless copy paper
- floor finish

PCBs continue to enter the environment.

PCBs entered the environment during their manufacture and during their use prior to the 1979 ban.

PCBs continue to enter the environment from:
• poorly maintained hazardous waste sites that contain PCBs.
• illegal or improper dumping of PCB wastes.
• leaks or releases from electrical transformers containing PCBs.
• disposal of PCB-containing consumer products into municipal or other landfills not designed to handle hazardous waste.

PCBs do not readily break down and remain for long periods of time, cycling between air, water, and soil.

PCBs can accumulate in the leaves and aboveground parts of plants and food crops. They are also taken up into the bodies of small organisms and fish.[73]

Health effects of PCBs.

PCBs are probable human carcinogens.

The EPA has determined that PCBs are probable human carcinogens. A number of epidemiological studies of workers exposed to PCBs found increases in rare liver cancers and malignant melanoma.

The PCBs that bioaccumulate are the most carcinogenic components of PCB mixtures.

The types of PCBs that tend to bioaccumulate in fish and other animals happen to be the most carcinogenic components of PCB mixtures. People who ingest PCB-contaminated fish or other animal products may be exposed to PCB mixtures that are even more toxic than the PCB mixtures contacted by workers.

The EPA has found clear evidence that PCBs have significant toxic effects in animals, including effects on:
• the immune system
• the reproductive system
• the nervous system
• and the endocrine system

The EPA points out that the body's regulation of all of the systems is complex and interrelated. And that as a result, it is not surprising that PCBs can exert a multitude of serious adverse health effects.

You might remember the story of the orcas from the beginning of this book.

"PCBs lower orcas' immunity to diseases, decrease sperm count and disrupt many hormonal, developmental and reproductive processes."

Studies in Rhesus monkeys, with immune systems similar to ours, have shown a number of serious effects on the immune system following exposures to PCBs. These include:

- reductions in the response of the immune system to an antigen
- decreased resistance to Epstein-Barr viruses and other infections[74]

Many who have been studying children with autism are aware of the immune system dysfunction. Many children on the spectrum appear to have persistent viral infections and persistent bacterial and yeast infections. There have also been reports of Lyme disease associated with autism.

Because there have been so many cases of viral and other infections, one theory has been, that it was these infections that have contributed to inflammation and the development of autism.

I think we will ultimately find that it is the poisoning by PCBs and other Persistent Organic Pollutants, that leads to, not only autism, but also to these infections. And that it is this poisoning that quite possibly has led to the explosion in the number of cases of Lyme disease.

Areas of the country that are hotspots for Lyme are areas of the country with heavy PCB contamination.

If you look at the areas of the country that are "hotspots" for Lyme,[75] you might find that you are also looking at areas of the country with heavy PCB contamination. This might help explain the high number of cases of Lyme in Wisconsin.[76]

The EPA further states that individuals with diseases of the immune system may be more susceptible to pneumonia and viral infections.

A recent study in humans found that individuals infected with Epstein-Barr virus had a greater association of increased exposures to PCBs with increasing risk of non-Hodgkins lymphoma than those who had no Epstein-Barr infections. PCBs affect the immune system.

More about Epstein-Barr Virus Infection and Autoimmune disease.

PCBs can lead to decreased resistance to Epstein-Barr infection. A recent journal article presented evidence that there is an association between an increased Epstein-Barr viral load and the development of autoimmune disease. It also proposed that deprivation of sunlight and vitamin D at higher latitudes facilitates the development of autoimmune diseases by further contributing to a CD8+ T-cell deficiency and further impairing control of EBV.[77]

In the young, PCBs are associated with deficits in neurological development.

Newborn monkeys exposed to PCBs showed persistent and significant deficits in neurological development, including visual recognition, short-term memory and learning. Studies in humans have suggested effects similar to those observed in monkeys.

Studies are ongoing to assess the effect on the endocrine system. PCBs have been demonstrated to have effects on thyroid hormone levels in animals and humans.

Elevations in blood pressure, serum triglyceride, and serum cholesterol have also been reported with increasing serum levels of PCBs in humans.

We have several studies showing a link between PCBs and diabetes.

I looked at some studies related to PCBs in previous chapters. There are several studies showing a link between PCBs and diabetes.

Just to put this in perspective, between 1980 and 2004, the number of Americans with diabetes increased from 5.8 million to 14.7 million.

The number of Americans with diabetes almost tripled in 25 years.

During that time period, the population of the United States increased from 227.23 million to 292.81 million. Obviously, the population of the United States did not triple during these 25 years.

We are seeing a significant increase in the number of children with autism, but we are also seeing a significant increase in the number of people with chronic diseases, including diabetes.

In a study of Adult Native Americans, exposure to PCBs and chlorinated pesticides was associated with the development of diabetes.

Another study looking at a possible link between diabetes and chlorinated compounds was carried out with Adult Native Americans. This was in the Mohawk nation at Akwesasne, which is a Native American population residing along the St. Lawrence River that separates New York State from Canada. This population is traditionally a fish-eating community. There are three aluminum foundries upriver from the reservation. PCBs were used as hydraulic fluids at all three facilities. When PCBs leaked, they contaminated the local environment and entered the food chain.

Mohawk adults who were 30 years of age or older, and who had resided at or near Akwesasne for at lest 5 years, could participate in this study.

In this study, elevated serum PCBs, DDE (dichlorodiphenyldichloroethylene), and HCB (hexachlorobenzene) were associated with diabetes. Showing an association with these chemicals, shows a possible link between PCB and pesticide exposure, and developing diabetes.[78]

The authors note that although the results do not establish cause and effect, there is a growing body of evidence that environmental exposure to persistent organochlorine compounds is associated with elevated incidence of diabetes. Elevated incidence of diabetes was found following dioxin exposure in Seveso, Italy. This was also found in a large study of workers exposed to dioxins during production of phenoxy herbicides and chlorophenol. Multiple other studies are cited that show a possible link between insulin levels and polychlorinated hydrocarbons.

Why are PCBs able to cause disease?

Many PCBs are considered to be endocrine disruptors. They appear to mimic a person's own hormones.

A possible mechanism by which PCBs may be able to mimic natural hormones, is through their biochemical structure.

The structure of a PCB is responsible for its recognition by cellular receptors. PCBs mimic thyroid hormones and other steroid hormones, including estrogen.

The toxic effects of PCBs appear to involve at least 3 types of mechanisms of action:

1. reversible interaction (binding) of the PCB with specific molecular sites, such as receptors, enzymes, etc.
2. irreversible covalent interaction (binding) between the PCB (or reactive metabolite) and target molecules (such as DNA and proteins).
3. accumulation of highly lipid-soluble, metabolically stable PCBs in lipid-rich tissues or tissue compartments.[79]

Are you eating PCBs?

Food samples from supermarkets in Dallas Texas were evaluated for PCBs as well as for perfluorinated compounds and organochlorine pesticide contamination. Six PCB congeners (six types of PCBs) of seven PCBs were found in salmon and canned sardines. PCB congeners were also found in hamburger meat, peanut butter and ice cream.[80]

Chapter 10:

Iodine

What treatment strategies are available for removing PCBs and other toxins from our bodies?

There is evidence that Insulin Resistance is playing a role in the cellular events that are contributing to Autism and Alzheimer's Disease. There is also evidence that chlorinated chemicals, such as PCBs and other polychlorinated compounds, may be contributing to the Insulin Resistance.

There is very little information in the literature suggesting treatment strategies for removing the toxins that are causing the cellular malfunction in the central nervous system.

Is Autism due to poisoning?

If Autism is due to poisoning, then removing the poison(s) may allow the brain to repair and to function correctly. Autism, as poisoning, explains a lot.

This explains what many parents have witnessed and reported. They report having a child with neuro-typical behavior and speech one day, that regresses and stops talking the next.

There is ongoing research regarding insulin resistance, hyper-insulinemia and the NMDA receptors.
This also fits the model when the onset is more gradual, that as the brain develops and there are more NMDA glutamate receptors, the poisoning becomes more apparent.

NMDA glutamate receptors are involved in new memory formation (learning) in humans.[81]

There is ongoing research looking at the links between: insulin resistance, hyperinsulinemia (elevated level of insulin) and the NMDA receptors.[82]

In my working model, the severity of autism is determined by the combination of genetics, environment, and nutrient status.
Remember, every child is born with a toxic load, some greater than others. Every child is exposed to additional toxins after birth, related to their environment (air, foods, water) and medical interventions (acetaminophen, vaccines, anesthesia, other medications). According to my model, the severity of autism is determined by the combination of genetics (ability to detoxify, NMDA glutamate receptors), environment (toxins), and nutrient status.

What role does iodine play in all of this?
If you thought that iodine was just for the thyroid gland, think again. Iodine is used to make thyroid hormone, but it is also found in other (non-thyroid) tissue as well.[83] About 30% of the body's iodine is found in the thyroid and in thyroid hormones. The remaining iodine is found in a variety of tissues, including mammary (breast) tissue, eye, gastric mucosa (stomach lining), cervix and salivary glands.[84]

I have come to realize that iodine may have another role, a new role in our modern, toxic, world.

I have seen children take iodine and show rapid improvement in symptoms.

I have seen a child take iodine and experience better focus, better interaction with family, and resolution of stimming. I have seen a child take iodine and go from being aggressive and stalking his siblings, to being kind and loving, engaging in play with his brothers. In some cases, the effect persists. In other cases, it appears to be temporary.

I think the difference has to do with the amount of the toxic load that is still present. In a child who has been "doing Biomedical" for a number of years, and has had a significant reduction of toxic load, the effects appear to last longer.

What is iodine?

Iodine is a halogen. A halide is a compound that contains a halogen. The other halogens are; chlorine, fluorine, bromine and astatine.

I think one of the things that iodine is doing, is that the iodine is displacing other halide-containing toxins such as PCBs and other polychlorinated chemicals. Iodine may also be displacing fluorine-containing compounds and bromine-containing compounds. It has been suggested that iodine also has a role in helping to remove heavy metals from the body.

Whatever it does, it does it quickly. But, as excess iodine is cleared from the body each day, it has to be administered daily.

How much iodine does it take?

It depends on the person. The dose may depends on the severity of the illness, which may be a reflection of the severity of the toxic load.

Is iodine safe?

There is continued debate within the medical community regarding side-effects and toxicity of iodine. There are three notable physicians who have treated hundreds of patients with "high-dose" iodine, and have information available in books and on-line. Guy Abraham MD, Jorge Flechas MD and David Brownstein MD.

David Brownstein, MD, has a book called, "Iodine, Why You Need It, Why You Can't Live Without It." Visit his website at www.drbrownstein.com to learn more about his experiences with iodine.

All three of the doctors have articles on the Optimox website. The research page is http://www.optimox.com/pics/Iodine/opt_Research_I.shtml

A review of some of the iodine research, as well as their own research, is in the article, "Optimum Levels of Iodine for Greatest Mental and Physical Health."

When you read this article, pay attention to Figure 1. This figure shows "Physiological and therapeutic ranges of inorganic Iodine intake, excluding drugs with iodine in their molecular structure."

This is a very interesting chart, showing recommended intake levels, actual dosages used in studies, where the physiologic range is, and the two areas of the therapeutic range - the area with no adverse effect on thyroid function, and the area associated with adverse effects on thyroid function.

Very high doses, in the "gram" range, have been used for some conditions, but these doses are associated with adverse effects on the thyroid.

Low doses, in the "microgram" range, will provide an adequate amount for the thyroid, but the dosing in the "milligram" range appears to be required for adequate iodine for the breast tissue.

Iodine and fibrocystic breast disease.

Dr. Flechas tells of his experiences in clinic with the article, "Orthiodosupplementation in a Primary Care Practice". In working with women with Fibrocystic Breast Disease, it was not until they reached a dose of 50 mg iodine daily, that they had full resolution of breast pain. On this dose, the findings of micronodularity, tenderness, fibrous tissue plaques, macrocysts and turgidity take almost a year to completely go away. Once these symptoms resolved, the women decreased their daily iodine dose. However, many continued to take 50 mg daily to decrease the chance of the cysts returning.

Prior to beginning iodine treatment with any patient, Dr. Flechas takes a full history and evaluates the patient for evidence of thyroid disease.

Anyone contemplating iodine therapy should be evaluated by his or her health care professional and have routine follow-up evaluation and testing.

Iodine and diabetes.

In this same article, Dr. Flechas tells of his first experience with treating a woman for Fibrocystic Breast Disease who also had insulin dependent diabetes. At the time of her diagnosis with the diabetes, her blood sugar was 1380 mg/dl. For the Fibrocystic Breast Disease, she began taking 50 mg of iodine daily. One week later, she had to begin reducing her insulin dose to prevent hypoglycemia. Four weeks later, she was completely off the insulin and with no dietary changes, her average random blood sugar was 98. Over the course of the next 2 years, she lost 70 pounds.

Can iodine help improve diabetes?

After this experience, Dr. Felchas did a study of 12 diabetics. In 6 cases, they were able to wean off of their diabetic medication and to maintain a HgA1c of less than 5.8, with an average random blood sugar of less than 100. The range of daily iodine intake in these patients was 50 to 100 mg. The other 6 patients were able to lower the total amount of medications necessary to control the diabetes.

How is the iodine improving the body's sensitivity to insulin and other hormones?
Dr. Flechas notes that with iodine supplementation, the body appears to become increasingly more responsive to thyroid hormones. One theory, is that iodization of tyrosine in hormone receptors normalizes their response to the corresponding hormone.

Does iodine help in the treatment of PCOS?
He further reports on 5 patients with PCOS. All were treated with iodine with resolution of the PCOS.

What about allergies to iodine? What about the Wolff-Chaikoff effect?
In treating over 1000 patients with iodine, he reports less than 1% have had an allergic reaction, usually hives. There were no cases demonstrating the Wolff-Chaikoff effect.

What is the Wolff-Chaikoff effect?
This is hypothyroidism induced by high levels of iodine. However, the effect is usually temporary. The effect has been noted to be prolonged in patients with chronic systemic diseases, euthyroid patients with autoimmune thyroiditis, and Graves' disease patients previously treated with radioactive iodine (RAI), surgery or antithyroid drugs. The effect has also been noted in patients with a history of postpartum thyroiditis, in euthyroid patients after a previous episode of subacute thyroiditis, and in patients treated with recombinant interferon-alpha who developed transient thyroid dysfunction during interferon-a treatment.[85]

Is there a link between iodine, thyroid and PCBs?

So, back to iodine, thyroid and PCBs. What is the link? I refer you now to a study looking at bottlenose dolphins near the Georgia coast, in an area heavily contaminated by Aroclor 1268, a PCB mixture. In this study, 26% of sampled dolphins have anemia. The dolphins showed reduced thyroid hormone levels. Total thyroxine (T4), free thyroxine (free T4) and triiodothyronine (T3) negatively correlated with PCB concentration measured in blubber.

NEGATIVE CORRELATION - The higher the PCB concentration, the lower the thyroid hormone levels.

Also, T-lymphocyte (immune cells, a type of white blood cell) proliferation decreased with blubber PCB concentration, suggesting an increased susceptibility to infectious disease.[86]

Low thyroid hormone levels, anemia, immune dysfunction linked to PCBs.

So, in these dolphins, we see low thyroid hormone levels, anemia, and compromised production of T-lymphocytes. This appears to be another case of a polychlorinated compound interfering with thyroid hormone production, and either directly, or indirectly (due to the hypothyroidism) affecting the production of blood cells (anemia) and the immune system.

Iodine and Autism.

James Adams, of Arizona State University, published a study showing low levels of iodine in the hair of children with autism. The autistic group had iodine levels 45% lower than for controls.[87]

Iodine was found to be lower in adults with Type 2 Diabetes.

In a study published in 2012, of adults with Type 2 Diabetes Mellitus (T2DM), we see evidence of a relationship between low urinary iodine and having T2DM. In the adults with T2DM, the concentration of urine iodine was significantly lower than in healthy controls. The level of urinary iodine negatively correlated with waist and hip measurements, glucose, insulin, HOMA-IR (calculated value indicating level of insulin resistance), triglycerides, angiotensin II and C-Reactive Protein.[88]

Hypothyroxinemia and Autism.

In a study of a mother-and-child cohort that included 5,100 women, the researchers found a consistent association between severe, early gestation maternal hypothyroxinemia and autistic symptoms in their children.[89]

Hypothyroxinemia. A common condition in pregnant women. It is characterized by low maternal free thyroid hormone (fT4) concentrations with TSH concentrations in the normal range.

Hypothyroxinemia is related to neurodevelopmental difficulties.

In the past, hypothyroxinemia was thought to be insignificant for mother and child. However, in findings published in 2006, a relationship was found between gestational maternal hypothyroxinemia at 12 weeks gestation and neurodevelopmental difficulties that could be identified in neonates as young as 3 weeks of age.

An evaluation of the data by the authors, showed that first-trimester maternal fT4, but not maternal TSH or fT4 later in gestation, was a significant predictor of neurodevelopmental scores.[90]

Agricultural pesticides and marginal iodine status may contribute to autism.

Kevin Sullivan, from Emory University, discusses the possible role of the interaction of agricultural pesticides and marginal iodine nutrition status as a contributor to autism spectrum disorders.

For pregnant women who have a marginal iodine nutrition status, the disruption of the thyroid system, *due to exposure to organochlorines (pesticides that are chlorinated hydrocarbons)*, could induce iodine deficiency and result in negative effects on the developing fetus. It is noted that the iodine nutrition status among pregnant women is marginal. Also, given the negative effects of a number of environmental chemicals on the thyroid, he notes the increasing importance of ensuring that all women have an adequate iodine intake.[91]

Environmental Factor - Polychlorinated toxins.

Genetic Factor - Detoxification capacity.

Nutritional Factor - Iodine deficiency.
Polychlorinated toxins, iodine deficiency and insulin resistance. All related. All contributing to our current explosion of chronic illnesses. All related to the multiple organ systems involved.

All related to the loss of the health of our children.

Chapter 11:

Colliding Worlds

Better living through chemistry.

Better living through chemistry. No one can deny that our world has changed dramatically since World War II. We have seen many advances in technology and have "toys" that we could only imagine when we were kids, watching the Jetsons and then Star Trek.

What many did not realize, was that there were changes going on in the world, outside of day-to-day awareness. Rachel Carson was one of the first to issue a warning, a warning that was largely ignored in the name of comfort, progress and profits.[92] As reported in a NY Times article, after the publication of Silent Spring there were personal attacks against Rachel Carson, accusing her of being a communist sympathizer. In a letter to her publisher, general counsel for a producer of DDT implied that she was some kind of agricultural propagandist in the employ of the Soviet Union and that her intention was to reduce Western countries' ability to produce food, to achieve "east-curtain parity."

Is there a link between the current extinction rate and our own health?

The myriad of chemicals that have made life easier, have had an impact on all life forms on this planet, including our own. There have been at least 5 major extinctions in the past. Now, many experts believe we are in the "sixth wave of extinction". This extinction appears to be of our own making and may be our undoing. Experts estimate that the current extinction rate is somewhere between 100 and 1,000 times higher than the background rate.[93] What many people have not realized, is that the loss of hundreds of species should have been a warning, a warning that our own species was being poisoned. This appears to be what has happened. We are poisoned. Our children are poisoned.

Is there a link between the health crisis of the orcas of Puget Sound and the health crisis of our children?

Each generation since World War II has seen a greater load of toxins. And the part of this story that is crucial to understand, is that the process affecting the orcas of Puget Sound, is the same process that is taking away our children, our next generation.

The orcas have the disadvantage of being bound to the toxic food supply. We have choices. We can educate ourselves and each other, to learn to survive in our now toxic world. A world where we face the loss of our pollinators. A world where eating fish is a calculated risk. A world where the advancement of medical science and technology for monetary gain and power has overshadowed the potential for good that this same technology could provide.

Putting autism and the explosion of other chronic diseases in the context of poisoning makes sense from a mathematical point of view. Random mutations or an autism gene does not. And when I say poisoning, this is not just the air pollution, not just the heavy metals, not just the PCBs and other chlorinated molecules we are now born with and continue to accumulate, but also the toxic chemicals in our foods, the medications to treat our symptoms, and the overuse of antibiotics and vaccines.

We are part of the planetary web of lifeforms.
We, as humans, are part of an intricate planetary web of lifeforms, all interconnected, and all supporting the life and function of others. As we have separated ourselves and tried to kill all pests and pathogens, we have been contributing to our own destruction.

Antibacterial soaps do little to protect us from germs but have introduced another toxin into our system. The chicken pox vaccine may have decreased the likelihood that your child will get the chicken pox (while introducing a dose of neomycin), but leaves your child vulnerable for a chicken pox infection later in life when it is actually most damaging. Babies now are born with much less protection from measles and whooping cough, due again to a short burst of immunity from the vaccine, that wanes over a period of years.

It is possible that we have supported a growing market for vaccines without adequate consideration for the long-term consequences.

Our natural world has collided with an increasingly toxic world.
Worlds have collided. Our natural world, a world with the potential for robust health, with adequate clean food, clean air, sunshine (yes, real sunshine), and community support of families. This world has collided with an increasingly toxic world, with rampant marketing of more toxic chemicals, resulting in escalating numbers of chronic diseases, widespread fatigue, inflammation and mental deterioration.

Hope.
But, there is hope. ACOG, the group of obstetricians and gynecologist, is beginning to sound the alarm on the role of toxins in personal care products.[94]

Toxins in personal care products are causing birth defects and developmental delays in the babies as they are growing in the womb.

I am seeing more dentists move away from using mercury in dental fillings.

I am seeing more and more physicians speaking out about the link between toxic foods and our ill health.

I am seeing more and more parents thinking about the safety of their children and the potential risk of vaccinations.

And I am seeing glimmers of hope in helping our children rid themselves of the fat-soluble toxins that have been so difficult to remove. Many parents working with Biomedical interventions have made enormous progress with dietary changes and nutrient supplementation, but for many, there has still been some areas of their child's health that has been resistant to improvement. I think that, with iodine, we have another tool to use. It may not be our final answer, but it is most certainly another great step to take.

I have seen many people control their insulin resistance, and the other conditions related to the insulin resistance, with a low carb diet. However, the insulin resistance, the point at the level of cellular function, is still there. Iodine, however, may be able to alter this insulin resistance. The clinical results of using iodine with diabetic patients certainly suggests that this is the case.

We now have some ways to measure PCB levels, including a measurement that reflects the level of PCBs that are stored in body fat, that can give us more clues regarding the role of iodine therapy.

One of the things (among many) that I don't know yet, is, when using iodine, are we helping to clear the PCB load, or simply removing the PCBs from receptors and carrier proteins temporarily.

Is there more I can learn about recovery?

Will I stop looking for anything else to help with recovery? No. Just as there are a combination of things making us sick, it takes a combination of things to help us recover.

Will an individual ever be clear of all toxins? No. I don't see any way possible for this to happen. When I look at the level of PCB and other POP contamination of the environment, and the bioaccumulation and biomagnification of toxins in our food supply, I don't think any of us can be completely clear of these toxins. However, we can certainly reduce our overall body burden and reduce what the next generation is born with.

Chapter 12:

Elephants All the Way Down

"And what does that elephant stand on? Why, another elephant, of course. It's just elephants all the way down."

Everyone thinks it is turtles, but it's not. It's elephants. Anyone that has read Terry Pratchett knows that the great turtle is carried on the back of 4 elephants, as it travels through the space of the multiverse.

Not just one elephant in the room, but two.
With each successive generation since World War II, we are seeing an increase in chronic disease and an explosion in the rates of childhood illnesses, including autism.

I think, that to stop this explosion and reverse our accelerating rates of disease, we have to acknowledge, not just one elephant in the room, but two.

One of the elephants has to do with the evidence showing a link between vaccines and onset of autism. We can deny it, try to shrink it, try to paint it invisible, but it is still there.

The other elephant, perhaps explains why the first elephant exists.

It may be that, injecting toxins and live viruses into healthy infants carries very little risk. (Unlikely, but for the sake of this particular argument, let's pretend that the risk is minimal.) The problem is, that all of today's children are, by definition, poisoned, and therefore, not healthy. The other elephant is the evidence that each successive generation is more toxic than the last.

We can deny the existence of these elephants and deny our children a chance to recover. Or, we can acknowledge that both of these elephants exist and then proceed to figure out how to live and survive in the reality of today's world.

Chapter 13:

Recovery Steps

There are steps we can take, for our own recovery and for the recovery of our children. If you have a chronic condition or illness, you may be able to improve your health by following some basic guidelines.

Step 1: Stop Poisoning Yourself. The next chapter will look at many of the different ways to reduce exposures to toxins.

Step 2: Nourish the Brain (and the Body). You are what you eat. All of the cells of the body are made of some basic building blocks. You get these building blocks from food. The more "real food" you eat, the healthier your cells. We'll cover this more in Chapter 15.

Step 3: Replace Nutrients and Remove Toxins. Our nutrients should come from the food that we eat. However, for severe deficiencies due to prolonged illness, or for increased nutrient need due to poisoning, I often use nutritional supplements. In Chapter 16, I'll take you step by step through a process of adding nutrients to help restore and support optimized health. Please remember that all medical treatment should be done under the supervision of your health care provider.

Step 4: Use activities and therapies to engage the brain and body. The brain and nervous system responds to movement, sound and visual input to "program" the brain and body to work together. When there has been a delay in development due to poisoning and/

or lack of nutrients, the individual has to go through all of the missed developmental steps to "catch up". Therapies include but are not limited to:

1. physical therapy
2. occupational therapy
3. hippo (horse) therapy
4. speech therapy
5. vision therapy
6. listening, including music, therapies

Chapter 14:

Stop Poisoning Yourself!

It is very easy to declare, "Stop Poisoning Yourself!" but in today's world, pulling this off can be a challenge. And in today's world, we can never avoid all the poisons. However, we can significantly reduce the amount of toxic chemicals that we are exposed to.

Step 1. Stop using poisons to clean your home.

One of the first things we can do is to look at all of the cleaning products in the home. Chances are, you have a lot of toxic chemicals just in the household products that you use. Fortunately, there are cheaper and much safer alternatives. There are a lot of nontoxic household cleaners on the market, but you can do a lot with baking soda and vinegar.

For information on household cleaners, I suggest you go to www. ewg.org. This is the website for the Environmental Working Group which has a data base, Guide to Healthy Cleaning, that looks at all major household products on the market. You can also find great information at www.healthychild.org, including information on using baking soda and vinegar as household cleaners.

When we did the big overhaul in our household, Amanda, my daughter who has 3 sons, did a lot of research.

Amanda and I were very impressed with the philosophy and products of a young company that was the brainchild of a teenager named Ava. The company had started with body care products and then later added household products and products for baby. We have also been using products from Celadon Road.

I like using the products from Ava and from Celadon Road because I know that:

1) I am getting nontoxic products.
2) I am supporting a small business that is supportive of nontoxic living.
3) the consultant is helping to educate others on creating a nontoxic home environment.

If you were given this book by a consultant for Ava or for Celadon Road, please go to her/his website, and/or contact her/him for more information on removing toxins from your home.

Step 2. Stop putting poisons on your body.

Just because there is not a "skull and crossbones" on your bottle of shampoo, does not mean that it is nontoxic. It is hard to believe that so many toxic chemicals have been allowed to be in our personal care products!

I will refer you back to www.ewg.org. This time, look at their Skin Deep Guide to Cosmetics. This is where you will find information on personal care products.

There are safer alternatives on the market, and recipes available for making your own. Additional information can again be found at www.healthychild.org. I also get personal care products from Ava and Celadon Road.

Antibacterial soap is harmful to you and is NOT effective at protecting you from harmful bacteria. Plain soap is best.

Do your research before you buy sunscreens. This is another line of products with many toxins to be aware of and to beware of.

And then there are the bug repellants. There ARE alternatives to DEET and permethrin. The EWG and Healthy Child websites can tell you more.

Step 3. Stop putting poisons in your mouth.

Many of the toxins that we have accumulated came from the grocery store. The chemicals that are used in the agriculture industry, the pesticides and herbicides, are poisons. This is why it is important to seek out **organic food** that has not been treated with toxic chemicals.

The growing number of farmers markets, and the increasing availability of organic foods makes getting quality, nontoxic food, more obtainable than ever before. Many people are also learning to grow some of their own organic food, even if it is in pots on the patio.

The Environmental Working Group has food guides to help you make the most of your grocery dollars. You can also find more information about nontoxic food at the Healthy Child website.

The more you get to know your local farmers and the farmers market, the better for you and the community. The more you obtain your produce and meats from local farmers, the more you know exactly what you are getting.

You should also be aware of the options you have when buying seafood. I recommend that you obtain the least contaminated fish so that you avoid feeding your family additional toxins.

The up-to-date information on seafood can be found at www.seafoodwatch.org. At this website, you can download a guide for choosing seafood, or, you can download their app for iPhone and Android.

Other toxins in our food, are the innocent-appearing things like artificial colors and flavors. Some of these are neurotoxins. It is best to avoid all artificial additives.

There are other toxins that you can avoid, including acetaminophen.

Acetaminophen has been used as an over-the-counter medication in the United States since the 1960s. It is used to reduce fever and relieve pain. The most common brand of Acetaminophen is Tylenol.

Once in the body, the acetaminophen is converted to metabolic byproducts which must then be cleared from the body. In the process of clearing the metabolic byproducts of acetaminophen, glutathione is used. Depending on the amount of acetaminophen being processed, glutathione can be significantly depleted.

Why we need Glutathione.

Glutathione is an antioxidant. It is the major endogenous (endogenous - made in the body) antioxidant produced in our cells. It can neutralize free radicals and can maintain vitamins C and E (also antioxidants) in their active forms.

Glutathione is used in many reactions in the cells. Every system in the body can be affected by the availability of active glutathione (reduced glutathione).

Reduced - a term used in chemistry that describes the "state" of a molecule. Glutathione in the _reduced form_ acts as an antioxidant. Glutathione in the _oxidized form_ does not function as an antioxidant. It must be regenerated into the "reduced" form to be usable again.

Glutathione can be depleted by acetaminophen. When completely depleted, the toxic metabolite formed by acetaminophen destroys the liver cells.

Glutathione is important for detoxification in the liver.

Some foods are toxic.

Actually, some foods are toxic for those who are chemical sensitive, but possibly not so toxic for those who are excellent detoxifiers. However, emerging research is indicating that when civilizations began eating grains, many individuals developed degenerative diseases. Those populations who changed to a grain-based diet had shorter life spans, higher childhood mortality, and a higher incidence of osteoporosis, rickets, and other diseases associated with nutrient deficiencies.[95] To optimize nutrient intake and reduce consumption of pro-inflammatory foods, removing grains from the diet can be helpful. We will cover this more in Chapter 15.

Step 4. Make your kitchen safe for food preparation.

The pots, pans and other cooking utensils should also be safe and nontoxic. Check out the Healthy Home Checklist at the Environmental Working Group website. The Healthy Child website also has information on cookware.

Step 5. Clean your water for drinking and cooking.

There are many water filters on the market. I use a ZERO filter and keep it in the refrigerator. If I drink bottled water, my top choice is Mountain Valley water in glass.

Step 6. As you replace furniture and/or remodel, choose non-toxic furnishings and materials.

Many modern building materials release toxic fumes and gasses. There are now low-VOC paints on the market. There are a variety of natural flooring materials that can be used instead of carpet.

Balancing the cost.

I know, that when I buy a Seventh Generation product, or a product from Ava or Celadon Road, I am spending more than I would spend on a grocery store brand. However, I am "voting with my dollars", sending a message about what I prefer to buy.

Voting with my dollars.

When I "vote with my dollars", I am also supporting a company that is working to reduce the toxic load of our planet. When I buy from an independent distributor (like Amanda!) of a conscientious company, I know that I am also helping to provide an income to our families and neighbors.

There are hundreds, if not thousands, of nonprofit charities. Many are operated by very sincere and dedicated individuals. Many, however, are not.

How can we support a strong, local economy with income for our citizens?

I believe, to have a strong, local economy, with income, not handouts, for our citizens, it is up to us to actually support each other's endeavors with as much dedication as we give to the global charities. The more that people have a livable income, the more people there will be supporting the charities.

I also believe, that we have been taught (misled?) to only spend money at big boxes, for the cheapest product available. We have been taught, that to buy a product from a local business, or a person in direct-sales, is foolish.

> *--- I wonder if this information came from the same people who packaged a bunch of chemicals in a pretty box and called it "food". --*

My point is if we are going to give our children any chance of having a livable planet we are going to have to work together and support one another.

We are going to have to support local farmers and local businesses.

We are going to have to care, at what cost in human lives, a product was produced.

We are going to have to care, at what cost in the strength and life of the food web, a product was produced.

We are going to have to care. To open our eyes and see that the world we are in, is a world that we, at some level, allowed to happen while we cut coupons, cut corners, and had no idea where our food and products were actually coming from.

Now, we have to care.

Chapter 15:

Nourish the Brain (and the Body)

JERF

Just Eat Real Food. If nothing else, if you make no other dietary changes, just eating real food, is a good idea.

Just Eat Real Food means that you only eat food that actually came from a plant, animal or fungus (think mushrooms), with no chemical additives.

The Just Eat Real Food diet should also **minimize**:

- agricultural chemicals
- animal products from animals that are fed toxins and raised in unhealthy conditions

Fats vs Carbohydrates and the risk of developing Dementia

A group of researchers from Mayo Clinic studied people at risk for mild cognitive impairment or dementia. The median age of the participants was 79.5 years.

The risk of developing Mild Cognitive Impairment or Dementia was elevated in participants with the higher percentage of carbohydrates in their diet.

The risk was reduced in participants with a higher percentage of fat or protein.

They concluded that a dietary pattern with relatively high caloric intake from carbohydrates and low caloric intake from fat and proteins may increase the risk of Mild Cognitive Impairment or Dementia in elderly persons.[96]

Diets to reduce inflammation and promote healing.

For optimal health, I encourage a diet that focuses on Real Food, but also minimizes inflammatory foods (including sugar).

The Paleo-type diet is a great starting point. Paleo means different things to different people, but there are some general principles that are helpful.

There is no "rule" in Paleo that makes it a high fat, low carb diet. However, many of the recommendations regarding designing your own Paleo-type diet, encourage people to choose higher fat and lower carbohydrate foods.

The book I recommend to learn about Paleo and dietary choices is:

Practical Paleo, by Diane Sanfilippo. You can follow her blog at balancedbites.com. You can also follow her on facebook.

If you have children, then I would also recommend:

Eat LIke a Dinosaur by the Paleo Parents. They also blog and have a facebook page. Elana Amsterdam, of Elana's Pantry wrote the Forward to Eat Like a Dinosaur. She, of course, also has a blog and facebook page.

Another favorite blogger of mine is The Paleo Mom. Sarah Ballantyne, Ph.D. (a.k.a. The Paleo Mom) earned her doctorate degree in medical biophysics at the age of 26. Visit her blog at www.

thepaleomom.com. She is also on facebook. She has a book coming out soon called **The Paleo Approach**.

Intensive dietary therapy.

When more intensive dietary therapy is needed, I will often use the Specific Carbohydrate Diet (SCD) and eventually advance to a Paleo-type diet. The difference is that the Specific Carbohydrate Diet begins with very simple, easy to digest foods. This is where I start when there is inflammation and dysfunction in the GI tract.

My resource for patients for beginning the Specific Carbohydrate Diet is:

www.scdlifestylebook.com

This book was written by two people who each had gastrointestinal disease and found their way back to health through the Specific Carbohydrate Diet. They take a person step by step through learning SCD, how to prepare foods, and how to advance the diet. It is slightly modified from the version by Elaine Gottschall, but I think the modifications reflect what we have learned since Elaine passed away.

They have a Quick Start Guide that is free, at:

www.scdlifestyle.com

When it comes to diet and turning your health around, you don't have to take my word for it. Just look at what Dr. Terry Wahls did to begin her recovery from MS.

http://www.thewahlsfoundation.org/

Her book that is coming out soon, is called:

The Wahls Protocol: How I Beat Progressive MS Using Paleo Principles and Functional Medicine

Chapter 16:

Replace Nutrients and Remove Toxins

Where to begin?

This is where it is so easy to quickly get overwhelmed. There are so many different vitamins, minerals and nutrients to replace and optimize. There are different methods for reducing the body's toxic load. But, where to begin? What all to take?

I tell people that there are many paths to regaining health. Most of these paths follow the same basic guidelines but with slightly different treatment plans.

I'm not here to tell you that I have the only treatment plan or that you should use my plan. I will tell you that it is important to find a plan and follow it as best you can.

The following information, like every thing else in this book, is for informational purposes only and is NOT a substitute for personal medical advice from your own physician or other health care professional.

Please consult with your health care professional for your personal nutrient supplement plan. When I am working with patients, I use an individual plan for each one. The following is a generic guide, but is not intended to substitute for, or be, medical advice.

The Rainbow Plan

Instead of numbering steps, lets use a rainbow. We'll begin at the "bottom" of the rainbow and work our way up, taking our time to understand what we are doing.

Consider taking at least one week with one step, before beginning the next step.

RED - Binding toxins.

One of the first things I said we needed to do was to stop poisoning ourselves. We also want to support the removal of toxins from the body. Two things that I know of that can be useful for toxin removal are bentonite clay and charcoal. Both of these have a negative charge and will adsorb toxins with a positive charge.

Your liver is working nonstop to remove toxins from the blood stream and release these toxins into the intestines for elimination from the body. However, some of the toxic material will be reabsorbed from the intestines, back into the blood stream.

Charcoal is a standard toxin remover that is kept in Emergency Departments to be used in cases of drug overdosing, accidental and otherwise. It is given orally and binds the toxic material in the GI tract, to prevent the absorption of the toxin into the blood stream. Charcoal adsorbs the toxin.

Adsorb - The "attachment" of molecules or atoms to a surface. Adsorption involves surface energy, such as opposite electrical charges.

Bentonite clay acts in much the same manner as charcoal. However, Montmorillonite clays, like the clay available as Redmond Clay, are the only bentonite clays with the ability to both adsorb and absorb.

Absorb - A fluid permeates or is dissolved in a liquid or solid.

The Redmond Clay also contains minerals that can be the beginning foundation of nutrient replacement.

The idea is to bind toxins in the GI tract to support removal of toxins from the body. It is best to give the charcoal or bentonite clay separate from medications or nutritional supplements.

Charcoal capsules can be opened to mix with water or juice or other liquid.

Mix one charcoal capsule or one teaspoon of bentonite clay with 8 ounces of liquid. Give this as separate as possible from nutritional supplements or medications.

Unless there is a reason to NOT use the bentonite clay, this can be given daily. The charcoal should be reserved for acute GI illness or when indicated by your health care practitioner.

Detoxification Baths

Another strategy for supporting detoxification is Salt Baths. Different types of salts can be used including:

- Epsom salts, with or without additional baking soda,
- Salt baths, with or without bentonite clay.

The Epsom salt baths may help increase the level of sulfate in the body and this can help with detoxification. Epsom salts also contains magnesium.

Sea salt baths may help with removal of toxins through the process of osmosis and diffusion. The toxins that are released from the body are pulled into the bath water.

These baths could be used on alternating days.

For each bath, add 1 to 2 cups of salts per tub of water. If you are adding baking soda to the Epsom salts add 1/4 to 1 cup of baking soda.

Do you have silver teeth?

If you have dental amalgams, those silver/mercury fillings in your teeth, I would recommend that you consult with a "mercury-safe dentist" in your area. This dentist can advise you regarding the risks and benefits of having these fillings removed and replaced.

ORANGE - Support the health of the GI tract.

Support the microbiome.
Inside our gastrointestinal tract is a fascinating world. This is the world of the microflora, the world of microbes that live in our GI tract and help maintain our health. The microflora contains both bacteria and yeast/fungi cells. There are more cells in the microflora than there are cells in your body.

The microbes in your GI tract help you digest food and absorb the nutrients from food. They produce vitamins and also interact with and support your immune system. The microbes produce short chain fatty acids that nourish both the microbes and the cells that form the lining of your intestines.

These microbes began colonizing your GI tract shortly after you were born. We add to this colony with fermented foods and with the microbes that naturally occur on our food and in our world.

In our quest to "Kill Germs", we have been killing our microbiome.
We damage this microflora with antibiotics, agricultural chemicals and with other toxic chemicals. The more we try to create a world without "germs", the more we damage our internal microbiome.

We change the balance of microbes by eating a diet high in sugars and carbohydrates. Artificial additives can affect the microbiome and some artificial sweeteners alter the pH of the GI tract and affect the microbial balance. When you alter the environment of microbes, they change and adapt and can actually change to forms that contribute to disease.

When you alter the balance of the microbiome, you are more susceptible to pathogens in the GI tract. One example of this is the overgrowth of Clostridium difficile that can occur with antibiotic treatment, leading to profuse diarrhea.

There are several strategies for supporting your microflora. Many people consume fermented foods such as sauerkraut (refrigerated, not the shelf stable variety), kombucha, kefir or yogurt. You can also take probiotics.

If someone has never taken probiotics, I recommend that they begin with a low potency, 1 to 5 billion CFU, and slowly increase the dose over time. The dose is generally individualized. For some, increasing the dose will help bring diarrhea under control. For others, increasing the dose will help bring constipation under control. If someone is unsure how much to use, starting with a low dose and supplementing with fermented foods is a good idea.

A note about Histamines.

Histamines are associated with allergic reactions and inflammation. However, it is possible to have an excess of histamines that is not allergy related. This excess will cause allergy symptoms and inflammation.

Histamines can be formed from some foods. Some types of gut bacteria are histamine forming. Other types of gut bacteria will break down histamines.

If you are having allergy symptoms or other symptoms of histamine excess, such as red ears and cheeks, then you should be more selective about your method for replacing the bacteria in your GI tract.

Kefir, yogurt and other cultured foods are high in histamines. These should be avoided until high histamine symptoms have resolved or significantly improved.

You should also choose a probiotic that helps to degrade histamines and does not promote histamine production.

YELLOW - Sunshine vitamin, vitamin D3.

If someone is deficient in vitamin D3, they will be taking a dose to help bring their level up within range. If you do not know your vitamin D level, then you could consider supplementing with the dose recommended by the Vitamin D Council.[97] However, if you have elevated blood calcium or any medical condition for which you take a medication, please check with your doctor before beginning vitamin D3.

These are the doses from the Vitamin D Council:

Infants - 1000 IU daily. Maximum daily dose is 2000 IU.

Children - 1000 IU daily per 25 pounds of body weight. Maximum daily dose is 2000 IU per 25 pounds of body weight.

Adults - 5000 IU daily. Maximum daily dose is 10,000 IU.

GREEN - Green foods!

Everyone loves green leafy foods! Not! But, many people like fresh smoothies which can be made with a little fruit and some vegetables.

Chlorella is a supplement that is concentrated green food.

Kale can be made into "kale chips" that I have seen even the most picky eater in the world consume in record time. Fresh kale tossed with coconut oil or lard, baked up crispy and sprinkled with sea salt and garlic powder is a great snack. Spinach chips, with baby spinach leaves, can be made in much the same way.

Amanda (my daughter with 3 sons) has been posting recipes on our blog. Here is the link for the kale chips. http://ourwellnessjourney. blogspot.com/2012/09/kale-chips.html. You might find some other helpful recipes on the blog as well.

Terry Wahls is an MD on a mission. She has been working on her own recovery from Multiple Sclerosis. She began with taking supplements to support mitochondrial recovery and then changed her focus to nutrient-dense foods. Take a look at what she eats every day to get an idea of what she sees as a healing diet.

http://www.thewahlsfoundation.org/

BLUE - Time for some B vitamins and additional supporting vitamins.

You have now seen the importance of vitamin B6 and vitamin B12. Folate, especially in the active forms, is also very important and works with the vitamin B6 and vitamin B12. Ideally, you want optimal levels of the vitamins, in, or with, a multiple vitamin that is "clean". In other words, a multiple vitamin that does not contain wheat, gluten, dairy, soy, sugar, or other inflammatory/toxic chemicals.

Now would be the time for patients to add a good multiple vitamin, and then after a week, add vitamin B6 in the active form (Pyridoxal-5-Phosphate), with magnesium.

After another week, they may add a sublingual vitamin B12 (methylcobalamin or a combination of methylcobalamin and adenosylcobalamin) 5000 mcg daily.

INDIGO - Add good fats.

If you have been working on dietary changes, you have probably already added some good fats to your diet.

Saturated fats from grass-fed beef and bison, pastured pork and free-range duck are essential to health. Saturated fats can also be found in butter, coconut oil and palm shortening. Additional good fats are found in nuts, avocado, and eggs.

You'll find some omega3 fats in the grass-fed meats. Cold water fish that are wild-caught in Alaska are a good source of omega3 fats. However, if you are allergic to fish and/or are having significant histamine reactions, fish and fish oil are not for you.

VIOLET - Iodine

The RDA for iodine appears to be inadequate for restoring and maintaining health. Please refer to the previous chapter on iodine for more information on taking iodine.

Additional nutrients and supplements.

Some other nutrients and supplements that I use on an "as needed" basis include:

- Glutathione
- GABA
- Melatonin
- Milk Thistle
- Glucoraphanin containing supplement (from broccoli sprouts).
- CoQ10 or a mitochondrial support formula.
- Bone broth (homemade)
- Gelatin (Great Lakes, green label)

Glutathione can support detoxification. Some people take this daily. Some use as needed, during a "flare".

GABA appears to support better focus and may have a calming effect.

Melatonin can support sleep onset.

Milk thistle can support liver detoxification.

Glucoraphanin is a component of broccoli and broccoli sprouts. Glucoraphanin can support antioxidant enzyme levels and support detoxification. Supplements made from broccoli sprouts can support intracellular levels of glutathione.

Bone broth supports healing of the GI tract and provides important nutrients for mitochondrial support (amino acids and minerals).

Gelatin provides amino acids to support tissue healing and also provides mitochondrial support.

Chapter 17:

Resources

How to begin the journey.

Beginning the journey to recover your health can seem like an impossible task. But, as the saying goes, each journey begins with one step. That's all any of us can do, just take one step at a time.

There are several resources mentioned already in this book, including books and websites for additional information. I think that you will find these resources helpful.

Finding Supplements

One of the major obstacles people face, with this journey, is determining what nutrients and supplements to take. I cannot give you specific medical advice, but I can give you access to some of the supplements that I recommend for my patients.

Finding nontoxic products for the home and for personal use.

Depending on where you live, and the stores in your area, this can seem like an impossible task. Even if you have health food stores in your town, not every product that makes it on the shelf is nontoxic. You still have to be a label-reader. Referring to the information from the Environmental Working Group and the Healthy Child website can be helpful, but I also realize that this may mean learning a whole new vocabulary.

A quick shopping guide while you learn the ropes.

I have set up a page on my website with some links. You can go there and follow a link to find supplements. As you learn your way around in the recovery world, you may find new resources that provide what you need.

My website is: www.betsyhendricksmd.com

Look for the "Zero Point" page to find the links for supplements and for nontoxic products.

Your best resource.

Your best resource on this journey, is other people who are also on this journey. One of the reasons for writing this book, has been to provide a beginning roadmap, a resource to get people started.

The information in this book is just the beginning of what you will need to navigate this new and toxic world. As I said in Chapter 14, we've got to work together to provide safe, sustainable communities. We have to work together and support one another.

This book is just the beginning of my task. My task is to use this book to bring the information to groups of people who can then work together to learn and use the material to recover and maintain health.

I will use this book in classes that I set up, but I will also talk to groups who are interested in learning and implementing this material.

My vision.

1. I will use this book in a presentation, to introduce people to the idea of finding health in a toxic world.
2. I will use an accompanying workbook to teach small groups, step by step, how to begin the recovery steps.

3. People who complete the small group curriculum, will then go on to teach new small groups.
4. We will continue to support each other and those we find who are interested in supporting their health and the health of their family and community.

Chapter 18:

The Last Word (for now)

Please keep in mind that I am presenting this information as I understand it. It is in no way a complete, absolute, authoritative, handed-down-from-above document. I, like everyone else doing this work, am constantly learning and adding to my understanding of our world and what has happened to us.

This work, this document, would not be possible without the thousands of hours that others have devoted to this field of inquiry. I am daily humbled by the dedication and passion of those working to bring information to light, in the face of constant adversity and harm.

I am sure that as I continue to study, I will revise and update my working model of how we are broken and how we repair. However, the basic framework for recovery has not changed over the years and is the basic framework that is used by many who are practicing Functional or Integrative Medicine. It is the basic framework that is used by those in the Healing Arts, utilizing natural methods of repair and recovery.

My hope is that this information will help many begin or continue their path of recovery.

Betsy Hendricks MD
Conway Arkansas
501-327-2967
www.betsyhendricksmd.com

About the Author

Betsy Hendricks is a mother of two grown daughters and grand-mother of three grandsons. She completed her undergraduate degree at the University of Central Arkansas in Conway Arkansas, where she graduated with Highest Honors in Biology. She then completed medical school at UAMS in Little Rock, Arkansas. This was followed by a 3 year residency program in Family Medicine, also at UAMS. She was Chief Resident during her third year of residency. After residency, she worked in the Department of Family and Community Medicine at UAMS, until she decided to go into private practice so that she could create a more integrative practice for her patients.

Dr. Hendricks created the Arkansas Center for the Study of Integrative Medicine. The principles of functional medicine are employed in the evaluation and treatment of her patients.

Dr. Hendricks was inspired to begin to work with children with autism by Jill James PhD of the Arkansas Children's Hospital Research Institute, as well as by some autism moms. Her initial studies took her down a path looking at the connection with yeast and autism, and the role of biofilm in concealing the yeast from detection and eradication, all within the context of the biomedical model. She presented the biofilm information to the Autism Research Institute Think Tank in 2008.

Although this path of study increased her understanding of the biomedical model of autism development and autism treatment, the drive to increase her understanding became personal with the births of her grandsons. With her increasing knowledge and understanding, the household underwent a transformation of diet and supplementation, as well as purging of personal care and household products with toxic ingredients. Amanda, the mother of the grandsons, researched products for the children and the household. She also developed creative recipes for ensuring adequate nutrition for each child.

References

1   The Killer Affecting Killer Whale Populations
http://science.kqed.org/quest/2011/07/19/the-killer-affecting-killer-whale-populations/
2   PCBs in Orca Whales, By Katy Califf
http://courses.washington.edu/z490/ed/PCBsinorcas.html
3   The dynamics of persistent organic pollutant (POP) transfer from female dolphins to their offspring during gestation and lactation.
http://www.nwfsc.noaa.gov/research/divisions/cb/ecosystem/marinemammal/pollutant.cfm
4   Colborn T (2004) Neurodevelopment and Endocrine Disruption. Environ Health Perspect. 2004 June; 112(9): 944–949. Published online 2003 November 17. doi: 10.1289/ehp.6601
5   Stern M (2011) Insulin signaling and autism. Front. Endocrin. 2:54. doi: 10.3389/fendo.2011.00054
6   Pollution in Minority Newborns: BPA and other Cord Blood Pollutants. Environmental Working Group.
http://www.ewg.org/research/minority-cord-blood-report/bpa-and-other-cord-blood-pollutants
7   Lau NM, Green PHR, Taylor AK, Hellberg D, Ajamian M, et al. (2013) Markers of Celiac Disease and Gluten Sensitivity in Children with Autism. PLoS ONE 8(6): e66155. doi:10.1371/journal.pone.0066155
8   Hadjivassiliou M, Grünewald RA, Davies-Jones GAB. Gluten sensitivity - Editorial: Gluten sensitivity as a neurological illness. J Neurol Neurosurg Psychiatry 2002;72:5 560-563 doi:10.1136/jnnp.72.5.560
9   Schmahmann JD. (2004) Disorders of the Cerebellum: Ataxia, Dysmetria of Thought, and the Cerebellar Cognitive

Affective Syndrome. The Journal of Neuropsychiatry and Clinical Neurosciences 2004;16:367-378.10.1176/appi.neuropsych.16.3.367

10   http://www.nlm.nih.gov/medlineplus/ency/article/007470.htm

11   http://www.nlm.nih.gov/medlineplus/ency/article/007472.htm

12   http://vsearch.nlm.nih.gov/vivisimo/cgi-bin/query-meta?v%3Aproject=medlineplus&query=ataxia

13   Windham GC, Zhang L, Gunier R, Croen LA, Grether JK. Autism Spectrum Disorders in Relation to Distribution of Hazardous Air pollutants in the San Francisco Bay Area. Environ Health Perspect 2006 September; 114(9): 1438-1444.

14   Hornig M, Chian D, Lipkin WI. Neurotoxic effects of postnatal thimerosal are mouse strain dependent. Molecular Psychiatry (2004) 9, 833-845.

15   Palmer, RF, et al., Proximity to point sources of environmental mercury release as a predictor of autism prevalence. Health & Place (2008), doi:10.1016/j.healthplace.2008.02.001.

16   Rossingnol DA and Frye RE, A review of research trends in physiological abnormalities in autism spectrum disorders: immune dysregulation, inflammation, oxidative stress, mitochondrial dysfunction and environmental toxicant exposures. Molecular Psychiatry (2011), 1-13.

17   Miller CS, Toxicant-Induced Loss of Tolerance - An Emerging Theory of Disease? Environ Health Perspect. 1997 March; 105(Suppl 2): 445-453.

18   Badawi N, et al., Autism following a history of newborn encephalopathy: more than a coincidence? Developmental Medicine & Child Neurology (2006), 48: 85-89.

19   Herbert M, Autism: The Centrality of Pathophysiology and the Shift from Static to Chronic Dynamic Encephalopathy. in Autism: Oxidative stress, inflammation and immune abnormalities. Chauhan A, Chauhan V, Brown T, eds., in press, 2009, Tayor & Francis/CRC Press.

20   The Killer Affecting Killer Whale Populations http://science.kqed.org/quest/2011/07/19/the-killer-affecting-killer-whale-populations/

21 PCBs in Orca Whales, By Katy Califf
http://courses.washington.edu/z490/ed/PCBsinorcas.html
22 The dynamics of persistent organic pollutant (POP) transfer from
female dolphins to their offspring during gestation and lactation.
http://www.nwfsc.noaa.gov/research/divisions/cb/ecosystem/
marinemammal/pollutant.cfm
23 Durkin MS, Maenner MJ, Newschaffer CJ, Lee LC, Cunniff CM,
Daniels JL, Kirby RS, Leavitt L, Miller L, Zahorodny W, Schieve LA.
Advanced parental age and the risk of autism spectrum disorder.
American Journal of Epidemiology, 2008; 168:1268-1276.
24 Kreesten Meldgaard Madsen, M.D., Anders Hviid, M.Sc., Mogens
Vestergaard, M.D., Diana Schendel, Ph.D., Jan Wohlfahrt, M.Sc.,
Poul Thorsen, M.D., Jørn Olsen, M.D., and Mads Melbye, M.D. A
Population-Based Study of Measles, Mumps, and Rubella Vaccination
and Autism. N Engl J Med 2002; 347:1477-1482 November 7, 2002
DOI: 10.1056/NEJMoa021134.
25 Heidary, Noushin; Cohen, David E. Hypersensitivity reactions to
vaccine components.
2005 Sep;16(3):115-120, Dermatitis.
26 WHO FOOD ADDITIVES SERIES: 51
NEOMYCIN (addendum)
First draft prepared by Mr Derek Renshaw
Food Standards Agency, London, England
Dr Carl Cerniglia
Division of Microbiology, National Center for Toxicological Research,
Food and Drug Administration, Jefferson, Arkansas, USA
and
Professor Kunitoshi Mitsumori Laboratory of Veterinary Pathology,
School of Veterinary Medicine, Faculty of Agriculture, Tokyo University
of Agriculture and Technology, Tokyo, Japan.
http://www.inchem.org/documents/jecfa/jecmono/v51je02.htm
27 Selimoglu E, Aminoglycoside-Induced Ototoxicity. 2007; 13, 119-
126, Current Pharmaceutical Design.

28   Owens, K.N, Cunningham D.E., MacDonald, G., Rubel, E.W., Raible D.W., Pujol R. Ultrastructural analysis of aminoglycoside-induced hair cell death in the zebrafish lateral line reveals an early mitochondrial response. J. Comp. Neurol., 2007, 502: 522-543.

29   GILBERT A. LEVEILLE, RICHARD C. POWELL, HOWERDE E. SAUBERLICH, and WILLIAM T. NUNES. Effect of Orally and Parenterally Administered Neomycin on Plasma Lipids of Human Subjects. Am J Clin Nutr 1963 12: 6 421-426

30   NEOMYCIN SULFATE tablet [Teva Pharmaceuticals USA Inc]. http://dailymed.nlm.nih.gov/dailymed/lookup.cfm?setid=777dbfab-f83e-4738-ae1e-78619a9f82a7

31   http://www.drugs.com/sfx/neomycin-side-effects.html

32   http://ods.od.nih.gov/factsheets/VitaminB12-HealthProfessional/

33   Bertoglio K, Jill James S, Deprey L, Brule N, Hendren RL. Pilot study of the effect of methyl B12 treatment on behavioral and bio-marker measures in children with autism. J Altern Complement Med. 2010 May;16(5):555-60. doi: 10.1089/acm.2009.0177.

34   Richard E. Frye, Stepan Melnyk, George Fuchs, et al., "Effectiveness of Methylcobalamin and Folinic Acid Treatment on Adaptive Behavior in Children with Autistic Disorder Is Related to Glutathione Redox Status," Autism Research and Treatment, vol. 2013, Article ID 609705, 9 pages, 2013. doi:10.1155/2013/609705

35   Rimland B, Callaway E, Dreyfus P. The effect of high doses of vitamin B6 on autistic children: a double-blind crossover study. Am J Psychiatry. 1978 Apr;135(4):472-5.

36   James B. Adams, Frank George, and T. Audhya. The Journal of Alternative and Complementary Medicine. January/February 2006, 12(1): 59-63. doi:10.1089/acm.2006.12.59.

37   http://www.cdc.gov/growthcharts/who_charts.htm

38   Miller VM, Kahnke T, Neu N, Sanchez-Morrissey SR, Brosch K, Kelsey K, Seegal RE. Developmental PCB exposure induces hypothy-roxinemia and sex-specific effects on cerebellum glial protein levels

in rats. Int J Dev Neurosci. 2010 Nov;28(7):553-60. doi: 10.1016/j.ijdevneu.2010.07.237. Epub 2010 Aug 5.

39   Nguon K, Baxter MG, Sajdel-Sulkowska EM. Perinatal exposure to polychlorinated biphenyls differentially affects cerebellar development and motor functions in male and female rat neonates. Cerebellum. 2005;4(2):112-22.

40   http://www.cochrane-net.org/openlearning/html/mod12-2.htm

41   Gardener H, Spiegelman D, Buka SL. Prenatal risk factors for autism: comprehensive meta-analysis. Br J Psychiatry. 2009 Jul;195(1):7-14. doi: 10.1192/bjp.bp.108.051672.

42   Paula Krakowiak, Cheryl K. Walker, Andrew A. Bremer, Alice S. Baker, Sally Ozonoff, Robin L. Hansen, and Irva Hertz-Picciotto. Maternal Metabolic Conditions and Risk for Autism and Other Neurodevelopmental Disorders. Pediatrics 2012; 129:5 e1121-e1128; published ahead of print April 9, 2012,doi:10.1542/peds.2011-2583

43   Fabíola Lacerda Pires Soares, Rafael de Oliveira Matoso, Lílian Gonçalves Teixeira, Zélia Menezes, Solange Silveira Pereira, Andréa Catão Alves, Nathália Vieira Batista, Ana Maria Caetano de Faria, Denise Carmona Cara, Adaliene Versiani Matos Ferreira, Jacqueline Isaura Alvarez-Leite. Gluten-free diet reduces adiposity, inflammation and insulin resistance associated with the induction of PPAR-alpha and PPAR-gamma expression. The Journal of nutritional biochemistry 1 June 2013 (volume 24 issue 6 Pages 1105-1111 DOI: 10.1016/j.jnutbio.2012.08.009)

44   E. Thiering, J. Cyrys, J. Kratzsch, C. Meisinger, B. Hoffmann, D. Berdel, A. von Berg, S. Koletzko, C.-P. Bauer, J. Heinrich. Long-term exposure to traffic-related air pollution and insulin resistance in children: results from the GINIplus and LISAplus birth cohorts. Diabetologia DOI 10.1007/s00125-013-2925-x

45   Chang JW, Chen HL, Su HJ, Liao PC, Guo HR, Lee CC. Simultaneous exposure of non-diabetics to high levels of dioxins and mercury increases their risk of insulin resistance. J Hazard Mater. 2011

Jan 30;185(2-3):749-55. doi: 10.1016/j.jhazmat.2010.09.084. Epub 2010 Oct 14.

46   Allen E. Silverstone, Paula F. Rosenbaum, Ruth S. Weinstock, Scott M. Bartell, Herman R. Foushee, Christie Shelton, Marian Pavuk, and for the Anniston Environmental Health Research Consortium. Polychlorinated Biphenyl (PCB) Exposure and Diabetes: Results from the Anniston Community Health Survey. Environ Health Perspect. 2012 May; 120(5): 727–732. Published online 2012 February 14. doi: 10.1289/ehp.1104247

47   Hirokazu Uemura, Kokichi Arisawa, Mineyoshi Hiyoshi, Atsushi Kitayama, Hidenobu Takami, Fusakazu Sawachika, Satoru Dakeshita, Kentaro Nii, Hiroshi Satoh, Yoshio Sumiyoshi, Kenji Morinaga, Kazunori Kodama, Taka-ichiro Suzuki, Masaki Nagai, and Tsuguyoshi Suzuki. Prevalence of Metabolic Syndrome Associated with Body Burden Levels of Dioxin and Related Compounds among Japan's General Population. Environ
Health Perspect 117:568–573 (2009). doi:10.1289/ehp.0800012 available via http://dx.doi.org/ [Online 10 October 2008]

48   Ten S, Maclaren N. Insulin Resistance Syndrome in Children. J Clin Endocrinol Metab 2004 Jun;89(6):2526-39.

49   Lim S, Ahn SY, Song IC, Chung MH, Jang HC, et al. (2009) Chronic Exposure to the Herbicide, Atrazine, Causes Mitochondrial Dysfunction and Insulin Resistance. PLoS ONE 4(4): e5186. doi:10.1371/journal.pone.0005186

50   Lee. Mitochondrial Dysfunction and Insulin Resistance: The Contribution of Dioxin-Like Substances. Diabetes Metab J. 2011 Jun;35(3):207-215. English.

51   Ruzzin J, et al. Persistent Organic Pollutant Exposure Leads to Insulin Resistance Syndrome. Environ Health Perspect 118:465-471 (2009).

52   Sima A.A.F. Encephalopathies: the emerging diabetic complications. Acta Diabetol. 2010 Dec;47(4):279-93. doi: 10.1007/s00592-010-0218-0. Epub 2010 Aug 27.

53 Rector RS et al. Mitochondrial dysfunction precedes insulin resistance and hepatic steatosis and contributes to the natural history of non-alcoholic fatty liver disease in an obese rodent model. J Hepatol. 2010 May;52(5):727-36. doi: 10.1016/j.jhep.2009.11.030. Epub 2010 Mar 4.

54 Wang, C.-H., Wang, C.-C., Huang, H.-C. and Wei, Y.-H. (2013), Mitochondrial dysfunction leads to impairment of insulin sensitivity and adiponectin secretion in adipocytes. FEBS Journal, 280: 1039–1050. doi: 10.1111/febs.12096

55 Maltin CA, Duncan L, Wilson AB.Mitochondrial abnormalities in muscle from vitamin B12-deficient sheep. J Comp Pathol. 1983 Jul;93(3):429-35.

56 Christine P. Stewart, Parul Christian, Kerry J. Schulze, Margia Arguello, Steven C. LeClerq, Subarna K. Khatry, and Keith P. West, Jr Low Maternal Vitamin B-12 Status Is Associated with Offspring Insulin Resistance Regardless of Antenatal Micronutrient Supplementation in Rural Nepal
J. Nutr. 2011 141: 10 1912-1917; first published online August 24, 2011. doi:10.3945/jn.111.144717

57 C. S. Yajnik, S. S. Deshpande, A. A. Jackson, H. Refsum, S. Rao, D. J. Fisher, D. S. Bhat, S. S. Naik, K. J. Coyaji, C. V. Joglekar, N. Joshi, H. G. Lubree, V. U. Deshpande, S. S. Rege, C. H. D. Fall. Vitamin B12 and folate concentrations during pregnancy and insulin resistance in the offspring: the Pune Maternal Nutrition Study. Diabetologia. 2008 January; 51(1): 29–38.
Published online 2007 September 13. doi: 10.1007/s00125-007-0793-y

58 Eoin P. Quinlivan. In vitamin B12 deficiency, higher serum folate is associated with increased homocysteine and methylmalonic acid concentrations. Proc Natl Acad Sci U S A. 2008 February 5; 105(5): E7. Published online 2008 January 30. doi: 10.1073/pnas.0711541105

59 Kaya C, Cengiz SD, Satiroğlu H.Obesity and insulin resistance associated with lower plasma vitamin B12 in PCOS. Reprod Biomed Online. 2009 Nov;19(5):721-6

60   E Setola, LD Monti, E Galluccio, A Palloshi, G Fragasso, R Paroni, F Magni, EP Sandoli, P Lucotti, S Costa, I Fermo, M Galli-Kienle, A Origgi, A Margonato, and P Piatti.
Insulin resistance and endothelial function are improved after folate and vitamin B12 therapy in patients with metabolic syndrome: relationship between homocysteine levels and hyperinsulinemia. Eur J Endocrinol 151 483-489, doi: 10.1530/eje.0.1510483

61   Spellacy WN, Buhi WC, Birk SA. Vitamin B6 treatment of gestational diabetes mellitus: studies of blood glucose and plasma insulin. Am J Obstet Gynecol. 1977 Mar 15;127(6):599-602.

62   Labadarios D, Rossouw JE, McConnell JB, Davis M, Williams R. Vitamin B6 deficiency in chronic liver disease--evidence for increased degradation of pyridoxal-5'-phosphate. Gut. 1977 Jan;18(1):23-7.

63   Şehnaz Bolkent, Özlem Saçan, Ayşe Karatuğ, Refiye Yanardağ. The Effects of Vitamin B6 on the Liver of Diabetic Rats: A Morphological and Biochemical Study. IUFS J Biol 2008, 67(1):1-7.

64   Emma M. Bingham, David Hopkins, Diarmuid Smith, Andrew Pernet, William Hallett, Laurence Reed, Paul K. Marsden, and Stephanie A. Amiel
The Role of Insulin in Human Brain Glucose Metabolism: An18Fluoro-Deoxyglucose Positron Emission Tomography Study
Diabetes December 2002 51:3384-3390;doi:10.2337/diabetes.51.12.3384

65   http://clinicaltrials.gov/show/NCT01767909

66   Craft S, Baker LD, Montine TJ, et al. Intranasal Insulin Therapy for Alzheimer Disease and Amnestic Mild Cognitive Impairment: A Pilot Clinical Trial. Arch Neurol. 2012;69(1):29-38. doi:10.1001/archneurol.2011.233.

67   Auriel A. Willette, Guofan Xu, Sterling C. Johnson, Alex C. Birdsill, Erin M. Jonaitis, Mark A. Sager, Bruce P. Hermann, Asenath La Rue, Sanjay Asthana, and Barbara B. Bendlin. Insulin Resistance, Brain Atrophy, and Cognitive Performance in Late Middle–Aged Adults.

Diabetes Care February 2013 36:443-449; published ahead of print October 15, 2012, doi:10.2337/dc12-0922

68 Konrad Talbot, Hoau-Yan Wang, Hala Kazi, Li-Ying Han, Kalindi P. Bakshi, Andres Stucky, Robert L. Fuino, Krista R. Kawaguchi, Andrew J. Samoyedny, Robert S. Wilson, Zoe Arvanitakis, Julie A. Schneider, Bryan A. Wolf, David A. Bennett, John Q. Trojanowski, Steven E. Arnold. Demonstrated brain insulin resistance in Alzheimer's disease patients is associated with IGF-1 resistance, IRS-1 dysregulation, and cognitive decline. J Clin Invest. 2012; 122(4):1316–1338 doi:10.1172/JCI59903

69 Suzanne M de la Monte. Brain Insulin Resistance and Deficiency as Therapeutic Targets in Alzheimer's Disease. Curr Alzheimer Res. 2012 January; 9(1): 35–66.

70 Edelson SM. The secretin story: still a promising treatment for autism. Autism Research Review International, 2008, Vol. 22, No. 2, pp 3 & 6.

71 E. W. Kraegen, D. J. Chisholm, J. D. Young and L. Lazarus. The gastrointestinal stimulus to insulin release: II. A dual action of secretin. J Clin Invest. 1970;49(3):524–529. doi:10.1172/JCI106262.

72 Dupre J, Chisholm DJ, McDonald TJ, Rabinovitch A. Effects of secretin on insulin secretion and glucose tolerance. Can J Physiol Pharmacol. 1975 Dec;53(6):1115-21.

73 Polychlorinated Biphenyls (PCBs), Basic Information. U. S. Environmental Protection Agency http://www.epa.gov/osw/hazard/tsd/pcbs/about.htm

74 Polychlorinated Biphenyls (PCBs), Health Effects of PCBs. U. S. Environmental Protection Agency http://www.epa.gov/osw/hazard/tsd/pcbs/pubs/effects.htm

75 Lyme Disease Date, CDC http://www.cdc.gov/lyme/stats/index.html

76 U.S. Files PCB Cleanup Lawsuit Against 12 Polluters of Wisconsin's Fox River. The United States Department of Justice. http://www.justice.gov/opa/pr/2010/October/10-enrd-1150.html

77   Pender MP. CD8+ T-Cell Deficiency, Epstein-Barr Virus Infection, Vitamin D Deficiency, and Steps to Autoimmunity: A Unifying Hypothesis. Autoimmune Diseases Volume 2012, Article ID 189096.

78   Neculai Codru, Maria J. Schymura, Serban Negoita, The Akwesasne Task Force on the Environment, Robert Rej, and David O. Carpenter. Diabetes in Relation to Serum Levels of Polychlorinated Biphenyls and Chlorinated Pesticides in Adult Native Americans. Environ Health Perspect 115:1442–1447 (2007). doi:10.1289/ehp.10315 available via http://dx.doi.org/ [Online 17 July 2007]

79   McKinney JD, Waller, CL. Polychlorinated Biphenyls as Hormonally Active Structural Analogues. Environmental Health Perspectives 102: 290-297 (1994)

80   Schecter A, Colacino J, Haffner D, Patel K, Opel M, Papke O, Bimbaum. Perfluorinated Compounds, Polychlorinated Biphenyls, and Organochlorine Pesticide Contamination in Composite Food Samples from Dallas, Texas, USA. Environ Health Perspect. 2010 June; 118(6): 796–802.

81   Rezvani AH. Involvement of the NMDA System in Learning and Memory. In: Levin ED, Buccafusco JJ, editors. Animal Models of Cognitive Impairment. Boca Raton (FL): CRC Press; 2006. Chapter 4. Available from: http://www.ncbi.nlm.nih.gov/books/NBK2532/

82   Eduardo D. Martín, Ana Sánchez-Perez, José Luis Trejo, Juan Antonio Martin-Aldana, Marife Cano Jaimez, Sebastián Pons, Carlos Acosta Umanzor, Lorena Menes, Morris F. White, and Deborah J. Burks. IRS-2 Deficiency Impairs NMDA Receptor-Dependent Long-term Potentiation. Cereb. Cortex (2012) 22 (8): 1717-1727 first published online September 27, 2011doi:10.1093/cercor/bhr216

83   Eskin BA, Sparks CE, Lamont BI. The intracellular metabolism of iodine in carcinogenesis. Biol Trace Elem Res. 1979 Jun;1(2):101-17.

84   Patrick L, Iodine: Deficiency and Therapeutic Considerations. Alternative Medicine Review, Vol 13, Number 2, June 2008.

85   Markou K, Georgopoulos N, Kyriazopoulou V, Vagenakis AG. Iodine-Induced hypothyroidism. Thyroid. 2001 May;11(5):501-10.

86 Lori H. Schwacke, Eric S. Zolman, Brian C. Balmer, Sylvain De Guise, R. Clay George, Jennifer Hoguet, Aleta A. Hohn, John R. Kucklick, Steve Lamb, Milton Levin, Jenny A. Litz, Wayne E. McFee, Ned J. Place, Forrest I. Townsend, Randall S. Wells, and Teresa K. Rowles
Anaemia, hypothyroidism and immune suppression associated with polychlorinated biphenyl exposure in bottlenose dolphins (Tursiops truncatus)
Proc. R. Soc. B January 7, 2012 279 1726 48-57; published ahead of print May 25, 2011,doi:10.1098/rspb.2011.0665 1471-2954

87 J. B. Adams, C. E. Holloway, F. George, and D. Quig. Analyses of toxic metals and essential minerals in the hair of Arizona children with autism and associated conditions, and their mothers. Biological Trace Element Research, Vol. 110, 2006, 193-209.

88 Al-Attas OS, Al-Daghri NM, Alkharfy KM, Alokail MS, Al-Johani NJ, Abd-Alrahman SH, Yakout SM, Draz HM, Sabico S. Urinary iodine is associated with insulin resistance in subjects with diabetes mellitus type 2. Exp Clin Endocrinol Diabetes. 2012 Nov;120(10):618-22. doi: 10.1055/s-0032-1323816. Epub 2012 Nov 30.

89 Román, G. C., Ghassabian, A., Bongers-Schokking, J. J., Jaddoe, V. W. V., Hofman, A., de Rijke, Y. B., Verhulst, F. C. and Tiemeier, H. (2013), Association of gestational maternal hypothyroxinemia and in-creased autism risk. Ann Neurol., 74: 733–742. doi: 10.1002/ana.23976

90 Libbe Kooistra, Susan Crawford, Anneloes L. van Baar, Evelien P. Brouwers, and Victor J. Pop. Neonatal Effects of Maternal Hypothyroxinemia During Early Pregnancy.
Pediatrics January 2006; 117:1 161-167; doi:10.1542/peds.2005-0227

91 Sullivan KM. The Interaction of Agricultural Pesticides and Marginal Iodine Nutrition Status as a Cause of Autism Spectrum Disorders. Environ Health Perspect. 2008 April; 116(4): A155.

92 Griswold E, How Silent Spring Ignited the Environmental Movement. NY Times (2012), http://www.nytimes.com/2012/09/23/magazine/how-silent-spring-ignited-the-environmental-movement.html?pagewanted=all

93   Ballantyne C. 10 Animals That May Go Extinct in the Next 10 Years. Scientific American (2007), http://www.scientificamerican.com/article.cfm?id=critically-endangered-species

94   ACOG. Environmental Chemicals Harm Reproductive Health. http://www.acog.org/About_ACOG/News_Room/News_Releases/2013/Environmental_Chemicals_Harm_Reproductive_Health

95   O'Keefe JH, Cordain L. Cardiovascular Disease Resulting From a Diet and Lifestyle at Odds With Our Paleolithic Genome: How to Become a 21st-Century Hunter-Gatherer. Mayo Clin Proc. 2004;79:101-108.

96   Roberts RO, Roberts LA, Geda YE, Cha RH, Pankratz VS, O'Connor HM, Knopman DS, Petersen RC. Relative intake of macronutrients impacts risk of mild cognitive impairment or dementia. J Alzheimers Dis. 2012;32(2):329-39.

97   http://www.vitamindcouncil.org/about-vitamin-d/how-do-i-get-the-vitamin-d-my-body-needs/

Made in the USA
Charleston, SC
27 April 2014